MORE PRAISE FOR DR. DINUBILE AND *FrameWork*

"No doubt about it, *FrameWork* is an important book that I know you will enjoy and find helpful on your road to optimal health, conditioning, and achievement. It's a must-read for anyone who cares about his or her body and wants it to last."

—Governor Arnold Schwarzenegger

"During my 21-year major-league career it was amazing to see the advances in training and medicine from the time I first made it to the big leagues in 1981 to the time I retired in 2001. Dr. DiNubile's book is a striking example of that and how a firm understanding of your body and how best to keep it in shape can enhance every part of your life. Having gone through my share of injuries, from bumps and bruises to a herniated disk, I wish that resources like *FrameWork* were available to me throughout my career."

—Cal Ripken, Jr.,
baseball's all-time "Iron Man," two-time AL MVP, perennial All-Star

"Dr. Nick has the uncanny ability to understand the language of the human body. He knows how it speaks. In the movie industry and in sports, the body is invaluable as an instrument. Dr. Nick is invaluable at keeping that instrument tuned to perfection. He is a healer of the highest order."

—M. Night Shyamalan,
The Sixth Sense, Unbreakable,
Signs, The Village

"*FrameWork* is an indispensable text that gives individuals essential advice and information on how to protect and enhance arguably our most valuable asset—the health and function of our musculoskeletal systems. Renowned orthopedic surgeon Dr. Nicholas DiNubile offers a wide variety of useful tips and practical guidance such as how to conduct a simple self-assessment of the condition of our muscles, bones, and joints, and, more importantly, how to properly exercise to safely improve our functional movement capabilities. At the American Council on Exercise, we were so impressed with the content in *FrameWork* that it is used as the core foundation of a continuing education course for our more than 50,000 fitness professionals. This book is a must-read for anyone interested in experiencing the joys of leading a physically active lifestyle and developing a body that's built to last a lifetime."

—Cedric X. Bryant, PhD, FACSM,
chief science officer, American Council on Exercise

"I have known Dr. DiNubile for many years, and his reputation as a specialist in sports medicine is legendary. Now he has compiled into book form knowledge accumulated from many years of working with athletes, which should enable even the nonathlete to achieve total fitness."

—Kenneth H. Cooper, MD, MPH,
founder, president, and CEO, The Cooper Aerobics Center

"This is the owner's manual that should have come with your body."

—Dr. Neil Liebman,
team chiropractor, Philadelphia 76ers

"Dr. Nick is a great doctor. He's not only an excellent surgeon but also an understanding, feeling practitioner in all musculoskeletal-related concerns. As he says, since we are living longer, this aspect of health care has surpassed the common cold for frequency of treatment. I am fortunate enough to have had Dr. Nick repair one of my knees. Being a good example of just the kind of extended-wear person Dr. Nick is talking about, now I am even more grateful to get advice from one of the brightest (and nicest) guys in the field on how to keep my frame working for me. I, like a lot of us who have borrowed time from science, can only very strongly recommend his words to anyone and everyone interested in keeping their bones working to their best potential as we gracefully glide, run, skip, bat, pole-vault, hike, or bike into our happiest days."

—William Hurt,
Academy Award–winning actor

"Dr. DiNubile is the master of preventative medicine for the musculoskeletal system."

—Wayne L. Westcott, PhD, CSCS,
fitness research director, South Shore YMCA, Quincy, MA

"*FrameWork* teaches you how to take optimal care of your body so you can enjoy both life and leisure more. For athletes, it's essential for a long healthy career."

—Jay Sigel,
U.S. PGA and U.S. amateur golf champion

"Dr. DiNubile's *FrameWork* provides cutting-edge information not only from a health and wellness standpoint but from an athletic performance aspect as well."

—Gary Vitti,
head trainer, LA Lakers

FrameWork

for the

LOWER BACK

A 6-STEP PLAN FOR A HEALTHY LOWER BACK

Revised and Updated—2nd Edition

NICHOLAS A. DiNUBILE, MD

with Bruce Scali

END BACK PAIN NOW!

RODALE

This book is intended as a reference volume only, not as a medical manual.
The information given here is designed to help you make informed decisions about your health.
It is not intended as a substitute for any treatment that may have been prescribed by your doctor.
If you suspect that you have a medical problem, we urge you to seek competent medical help.

The information in this book is meant to supplement, not replace, proper exercise training. All forms of exercise pose some inherent risks. The editors and publisher advise readers to take full responsibility for their safety and know their limits. Before practicing the exercises in this book, be sure that your equipment is well-maintained, and do not take risks beyond your level of experience, aptitude, training, and fitness. The exercise and dietary programs in this book are not intended as a substitute for any exercise routine or dietary regimen that may have been prescribed by your doctor. As with all exercise and dietary programs, you should get your doctor's approval before beginning.

Mention of specific companies, organizations, or authorities in this book does not imply endorsement by the author or publisher, nor does mention of specific companies, organizations, or authorities imply that they endorse this book, its author, or the publisher.

Internet addresses and telephone numbers given in this book were accurate at the time it went to press.

FrameWork and Active for Life are registered trademarks of Nicholas A. DiNubile, MD.

2nd edition published March, 2010 by Rodale Inc.

Rodale books may be purchased for business or promotional use or for special sales. For information, please write to:

Special Markets Department, Rodale, Inc., 733 Third Avenue, New York, NY 10017
Printed in the United States of America

Rodale Inc. makes every effort to use acid-free ♾, recycled paper ♻.

Photographs by John Hamel

Book design by Christina Gaugler

Library of Congress Cataloging-in-Publication Data

DiNubile, Nicholas A.
  Framework for the lower back : a 6-step plan for a healthy lower back / Nicholas A. DiNubile ; with Bruce Scali.
      p.   cm.
  Includes index.
  ISBN-13 978–1–60529–197–0 pbk.
  1. Backache—Exercise therapy.   2. Physical fitness.   I. Scali, Bruce.   II. Title.
RD771.B217D56   2009
617.5'64062—dc22   2009045641

Distributed to the trade by Macmillan
2   4   6   8   10   9   7   5   3   1   paperback

We inspire and enable people to improve their lives and the world around them

For more of our products visit **rodalestore.com** or call 800-848-4735

To my dream team:
Marybeth, Emily, and Dylan

ACKNOWLEDGMENTS

It would be almost impossible to acknowledge the many individuals who have helped influence and shape my thoughts and philosophy as expressed in *FrameWork for the Lower Back*. Teachers, medical colleagues, patients, and friends, in the gym or on the field, have all had an impact for which I am grateful.

I would also like to extend my sincere gratitude to the following individuals: Arnold Schwarzenegger for his friendship and inspiration over the years and also "the gang" at Oak Productions, especially Lynn Marks; David Caruso, my friend and partner in creating innovative health solutions through technology; Lois de la Haba, my agent, who believed in me and this project from the very beginning; Bruce Scali for his talent, professionalism, and collaboration; the top-notch, enthusiastic team at Rodale, including Karen Rinaldi, Chris Krogermeier, Colin Dickerman, Courtney Conroy, and also John Hamel, Troy Schnyder, Christina Gaugler, Lois Hazel, Joanna Williams, and Adrienne Bearden-Gardner; Joe Kelly, whose images grace the pages of this book; Roger Schwab for his friendship and thought-provoking discussions and state-of-the-art workouts and facility at Main Line Health and Fitness; the Philadelphia 76ers and Pennsylvania Ballet, two first-class organizations I've had the pleasure to work with over the years and where I have learned firsthand the extraordinary capabilities of the human body and that given the right circumstances, healing can indeed be accelerated; Frank Nein for his help and support in cyberspace, especially at www.drnick.com; the many physicians and health care professionals who contributed their thoughts, philosophy, and expertise found within the pages of this book; my dedicated staff, Mary Moran and Barb De Jesse; and most importantly, my loving, supportive family—Marybeth, my wife and creative advisor, and my children, Emily and Dylan, who inspire me every single day.

CONTENTS

PREFACE

There's good news and there's bad news on the health care front: We're living a lot longer (life expectancy has doubled over the last hundred or so years, and the curve is still decidedly upward), but, as I've said before and never tire of saying, we've outlived the warranties on our bodies—our frames, if you will. The simple truth is evolution doesn't work very fast; it takes its sweet time to catch up, and the structure that was perfectly fine for an average 40-year life span a century ago isn't exactly up to snuff now.

Any machine, including the human one, will lose efficiency and break down at some point. Of all the people who have ever lived past the age of 65, two-thirds are alive today, so it's no surprise that musculoskeletal ailments leapfrogged the common cold in 2004 as the number-one reason for doctor visits. Problems with muscles, bones, and joints fill many physicians' schedules, driven in no small measure by arthritis in all of its forms. Lower back injury is the most frequent claim for those out on workers' compensation, and lower back pain is at or near the top of the musculoskeletal list for everyone else, too.

Including me.

You see, when I was a little younger, I sustained an injury that reminds me to this day of the one spent horsing around on a beach, when I got tackled and my back was wrenched in a way it wasn't designed to handle. I sucked it up then, I sucked it up later on, and there are plenty of days now when I suck it up and carry on—just as millions of others who have had a similar experience do.

I'm sure an MRI would reveal a bulging disk or some other frame irregularity that would explain the tightness and aches that visit me from time to time, but I never saw much point in undergoing that inconvenience and expense. Why? Because just about everyone—especially an orthopaedic surgeon like me—knows there isn't a surgical option that would apply to my circumstance. Even if back procedures were more applicable than

BACKBOARD

Lesson: Active for Life

Flexibility

Strength

Durability

Balance

they are (much more on this in Step 2), my condition doesn't justify going under the knife. Also, although MRIs and other sophisticated tests can provide a lot of information, in most instances, that information does not alter the approach that people should take to manage their lower back problems. It's likely that if you have a back problem, it doesn't call for surgery either.

The overwhelming majority of back conditions don't require surgery.

The good news is you don't have to live with chronic or occasional pain, or the perpetual compromised mobility and accompanying concessions that have become so routine that you don't even think about them anymore. Let me assure you that if you take the steps in this book, you'll reduce, if not elimi-

nate, back pain episodes; you'll be able to do a lot more than you're doing now; and you'll feel a whole lot better. Like I do.

If you're not one of the millions who negotiate back issues on a regular basis, then you opened this book because you know one or more of those people and want to avoid similar travails, or you've had a minor issue that you'd prefer to avoid in the future. Or maybe you're just the proactive sort who wants to focus on an area that's been missing from your regular exercise routine. No matter what brought you here, it's all about getting more enjoyment day to day.

"ACTIVE FOR LIFE"

Whatever shape you're in now, it can be better. You can move about better, you can recreate better, you can have a better foundation for later years. Bottom line? You can extend that warranty on your frame. How?

With an intention to do it and a commitment to regular exercise. It's all about mindset and movement.

If you're pondering how you could even consider a back program when just getting through a day without causing additional harm to yourself is an accomplishment, fear not. Whatever shape you're in, if you follow these six steps, you'll be stepping a lot more lively from then on.

A couple of years ago, I wrote *FrameWork*, a program that addressed all of the body's muscles, bones, and joints—everything you need to live life to the fullest. One of its keys for developing and keeping a healthy frame was building core strength. Your core is not just six-pack abs; it's your back muscles, deep abdominals, oblique muscles, hips, and pelvis, and if we take a journey to the epicenter of the core, we're talking about the center of rotation of your body—your

BACK STORY

The benefit of activity—both mental and physical—to my stiff, achy back was driven home on an exceptionally busy surgical day several years ago. I was distracted by my barking back, and it was one of those "suck it up" times I referenced earlier. I really didn't have the option of not showing up and standing for 7 grueling hours. So I soldiered on—and got an interesting back lesson.

Orthopaedic surgery requires precision, and that requires concentration. When one steps into the OR, one's mind focuses solely on the task at hand. That day, during a short break after a few hours in the surgery suite, I was pleasantly surprised to realize that my back wasn't barking anymore. In fact, it felt pretty darn good.

Out of necessity, I'd put my aches out of my mind, and I had done all of the turns, bends, and neck movements required to operate. It turned out to be a good day for my patients, and a good one for me, too.

By "letting go" of my pain—or at least putting it on hold for a while and focusing on something else much more important, my body had a chance to correct things. This is something I have seen and experienced over and over. And it is one of the reasons that sitting around focusing on pain, and what you *can't* do, can be very counterproductive for people who suffer from back pain, and why work can sometimes be curative. I believe the mind, what I call the executive suite of the body, can at times interfere with your body's ability to self-correct certain ailments. The mind can reinforce unwanted patterns and sometimes just needs to be distracted a little.

spine. You can't rotate without it, and you're going to rotate it whether your back hurts or it doesn't (unless, of course, you plan to stay immobile indefinitely).

Sedentary is not an option.

Fact is, sedentary is not an option for anyone. One of the conclusions of the *Surgeon General's Report on Physical Activity and Health* a few years back, that I was honored to contribute to, was that being idle is as dangerous for your health as smoking a pack of cigarettes a day. Other research is pouring in about the role of exercise in back pain; its conclusions, incorporated here, might startle you.

You've got to be active for life, yes, but we all know the body is not always cooperative—something or other gets in the way. Among the limiting factors is a musculoskeletal ailment, whether it's present now or on the horizon, with pain in all of its expressions. It's one of the biggest excuses why people don't do things or can't do things.

Being active for life requires a frame that is flexible, strong, durable, and balanced. It's all well and good to have "chiseled muscles" or advanced running capability, but if your entire frame isn't in shape and balanced,

you're a candidate for aches and pulls and sprains, for joint dysfunctions and arthritis and disk problems, for diminished mobility. Being active for life also means being pain free, or at least in pain "health"—able to live with it and move around in spite of it. (This is where your eyes will open wide when you discover how different—and better—your life is after you pay a little attention to your lower back, spending 20 to 30 minutes three times a week doing some simple lower back exercises. Everyone, especially those with pain and impairment, will benefit from the controlled, targeted routine in these pages.)

A lot of people come into my office and say, "I think I pulled a muscle in my butt or hamstring." If you're really young, you can pull muscles, but if you're getting aches and pains, they are usually messages being sent from deeper in the body outward. If you're hurting now in the back or pelvis or buttock area, the lower back program herein will help you unwind it.

And if you're in great shape now, it will ensure you stay that way. The FrameWork approach—self-test, core strength, flexibility, aerobic fitness, active rest and recovery, nutrition, and the mind-body connection—is all here to address lower back health. Specifics on the latter four topics are included in Step 4 because they are vital to consider as you implement your lower back exercise program. The "meat on the bones," if you will, of lower back health—general information, self-assessment, exercises, and pain management—is presented in the five other essential steps for a healthy back.

THE MYTHS OF BACK PAIN

As time goes on and our body of knowledge increases, we are able to dispel some common notions about pain and its treatment. At the top of this list is an assumption that people who have jobs that require them to use their backs like a crane, such as ditchdiggers, firefighters, and dockworkers, are the ones most susceptible to back injury. As we touched on earlier, the data is showing that those with a sedentary lifestyle, such as truck drivers and office personnel, may actually be at equal risk. And, as you will soon see, anyone experiencing heightened stress is set up for a back ailment.

Next, back pain isn't solely the result of a back injury. Improper exercise, sudden twists and turns and bends, shoes, and the natural aging process contribute to the growing number of people who suffer from back pain. Also, genetics can be a factor. Unfortunately, the

BACKBOARD

Lesson: Back Pain Myths

Strenuous labor is much riskier than sedentary employment.

Injury is sole cause.

Long bed rest is always best treatment.

Surgery is inevitable.

Back surgery is dangerous and doesn't work.

best advice I can give you in that regard is to "choose your parents wisely."

It is simply untrue that bed rest is always the best treatment for serious back pain.

Another myth—that extended bed rest is the best treatment for back pain—is of particular import to the program in these pages. A day in bed, or restricted activity, is a reasonable first prescription, but we now know that an extended immobile period weakens muscles and joints and actually extends the time that pain is felt. We know that most pain will subside on its own if you move about prudently right away and exercise moderately and properly as soon as possible.

BACK STORY

My wife is extremely fit, and she was extremely fit throughout her pregnancies. When she was delivering the last time, I remember the nurse saying to her, "I can't believe this—we can see your abs! You're in better shape than us and you're delivering!"

After every delivery, my extremely fit wife was still challenged in a huge way. We aren't the type who has somebody come in to watch our kids, so she stayed at home. It wasn't easy for her to get out to the gym, and she was usually so tied up and exhausted that working out at home wasn't much of an option either. When I came home from my long workday, she just wanted to rest; rehab, let alone her usual exercise program, was far from her mind. I learned firsthand the challenges women face trying to be fit *after* a new baby arrives.

We've been very fortunate that my wife never had any major back problems; but, to this day, when her back acts up a bit, she'll say it feels like it did when she was pregnant.

Closely related to this idea is the belief that back pain means surgery sooner or later. Wrong again. Most pain is the result of muscle strains, spinal wear and tear, and arthritis, and most disk problems and their associated pain can't be solved with a scalpel. Pain does respond, however, to a whole series of first aid alternatives that you can administer on your own. (Much more on this later on.)

The scariest myth is that back surgery is more dangerous than other major procedures, and doesn't work to boot. That isn't the case at all, and it does a disservice to the thousands of people who are at the point where there is no other option, when all conservative treatments have been tried without lasting success. Having said that, let me emphasize that the entire FrameWork philosophy is geared to keeping an OR date off the calendar—forever.

There are myths about pain, but pain itself is real enough. We are going to cover that—where it comes from and why—and what you can do about it to live better.

A PREGNANT PAUSE

Women comprise half of the population, and a large majority have been or will be pregnant at one time or another, an experience that actually consumes more than a year of their lives. There isn't enough attention paid to the fitness needs of millions of women who bring our precious children into the world. You'd have to search high and low to find anything written about how they should prepare for, and recover from, delivery. I always say (women love this) that if men were to go through that, there would be a whole program afterward, an entire manual to get back in shape as soon as possible. For women, men (and too many doctors) think, "It's okay, once you have the baby, you'll be fine, and all of this will go away."

But it doesn't, really. Pregnancy creates postural changes; many women just lean back to make up for the weight increase in front rather than building the strength to keep a better posture. After delivery, not only do you have less time to work out, but your sleep is erratic, you're carrying around significant additional weight (aka your new baby) in odd positions, and you're bending, lifting, and twisting more. These BLTs, as I refer to them, are part of Step 1 in your program for lower back health. Pregnancy also causes sleep disturbance and its attendant drag on health, especially back health. This is why some questions about it are included in the self-assessment part of all FrameWork programs.

I always tell women who are planning to get pregnant that it's like training for an athletic event—they should try to get fit, be fit, and then stay fit for the duration. There are plenty of things you can do *before* you get pregnant, during the first trimester, and after you deliver to restore your frame quickly. (If you're pregnant now and have never exercised, it's not time to start.) In fact, it is always prudent to consult with your doctor before embarking on any new exercise program, most especially in pregnancy cases.

If you're pregnant now, pay close attention to the posture and lifting recommendations in Step 1, and talk to your doctor about the back exercises in Step 5 that are appropriate in many cases. Ask him or her about some weight training, too—that shouldn't be automatically ruled out. Rather, it can be extremely helpful.

It's all about staying fit during a wonderful experience that nonetheless takes a toll on your body (a toll that increases with each subsequent pregnancy). It's about staying strong for the demands placed upon your frame (before, during, and after) and reducing the vulnerability to back pain inherent in childbearing.

It used to be an absolute no-no to exercise

during pregnancy; now, from an orthopaedic standpoint, it's an absolute yes-yes. As more medical professionals shed light on this issue, fewer women are left far behind after delivery.

FRAMEWORK RECAST

Your program for lower back health is comprehensive, but simple enough to implement and stick to. This FrameWork approach, richly enhanced by contributions from a few prominent doctors who specialize in the spine and were kind enough to contribute some of their hard-won knowledge, extends the usefulness and enjoyment of a critical part of your body. A part that is the keystone of your entire frame.

The first step in your FrameWork Lower Back Program—Think "Back"—is a short primer on the back's anatomy and biomechanics, and it includes a survey of the potential weak links that cause back problems. Step 2, Your Out-of-Whack Back, addresses back ailments, how to differentiate between pain and injury and recognize when professional help is called for, and how you can treat minor back ailments right in your own home.

Step 3 is Watch Your Back—Self-Test, where you'll answer a battery of questions and try some simple exercises to assess the status of your lower back. You'll identify those weak links that are uniquely yours as a result of your medical history, lifestyle, and current physical condition.

Back to the Start is Step 4—a few critical considerations before you dive into the lower back workouts in Step 5, Back in Shape. Everyone will start at the beginner level there, and you'll move up when you're ready for the next challenge.

If all of the benefits of exercise could be packaged in a single pill, it would be the most prescribed medication in the world.

The last step, Back Talk, is an in-depth discussion of pain and its management, and, even if you aren't in serious pain now, it will be invaluable if you join the ranks of those afflicted down the road. All of the best modalities and alternatives for treatment are covered, and the latest information and advisories related to surgical options are included.

It has been said, "If all of the benefits of exercise could be packaged in a single pill, it would be the most prescribed medication in the world." Studies are now proving that some genetic predispositions actually get turned on with exercise, so schedule regular periods for it. Get the PDA out, slap a reminder on the refrigerator or your desk, and block off time for the workouts your frame is crying out for.

You simply must make time for exercise. It is a wise investment of your valuable time, and it will pay huge dividends. As my good friend Arnold Schwarzenegger says, "Every hour you spend in the gym is one less hour you'll have to sit in the doctor's office." As usual, Arnold is right on with that very insightful message.

The FrameWork lower back routines will improve your range of motion, build core strength, and complement fitness in other areas of your body. You'll also note performance improvements in the sports you enjoy, such as golf and tennis, as your core is the center of the athlete within you. Make them a regular part of your (active) life because, just like any other prescription, the positive effects of exercise wear off over time.

IT COMES DOWN TO YOU

Changes in your body are inevitable; problems aren't. There's no guarantee that I have all of the answers for every case of back pain, and if you have a problem, chances are that if a board of representatives from every medical specialty consulted on your case, they wouldn't come up with all of them either. Why? Because *you* are part of the solution to any health issue you face. That's the answer I know that applies to everyone.

You have desires and expectations for the best of health, but you've got responsibilities in securing and maintaining it, too. Being lean and beautiful on the outside isn't enough. You've got to have a structure that's going to support you for the long haul, including a spine that's in good working order. That means getting and staying active no matter what your circumstances are. Beating back pain often requires an adjustment—sometimes it is a chiropractic one; more often it is a mind-set one. You can circumvent lower back problems, or prevent them, with the six essential steps presented in these pages, which are the right approach in every case. They're a key to healthy, active aging.

People who do more live longer. Bridge the gap between longevity and durability—get in the best shape you can, and give your frame every chance to resist breakdown or recover better from disease or injury.

It's in your hands, and it starts right now.

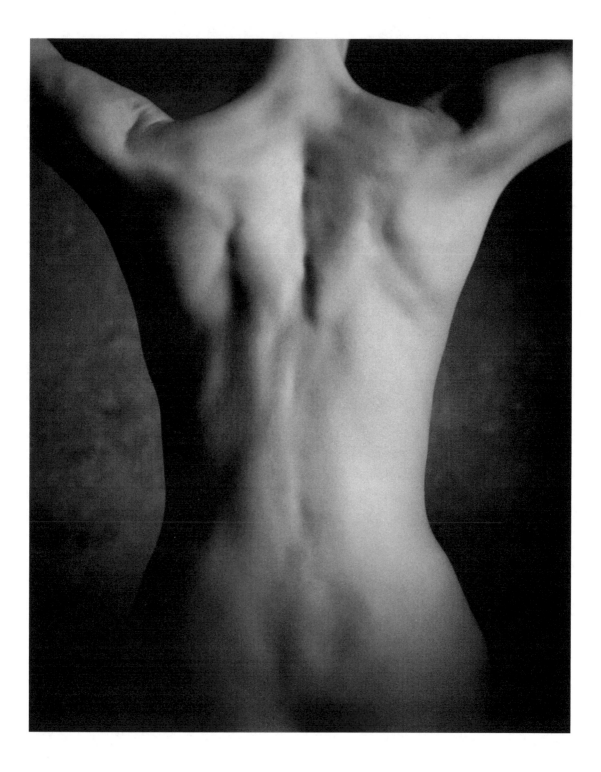

Think "Back"

Roger Schwab, founder of Main Line Health & Fitness in a Philadelphia suburb, is an oft-requested personal trainer for top U.S. athletes, and the provider of a first-rate exercise facility. What's really special about Roger is his innovative work in establishing Main Line Medical Exercise, a facility that incorporates the latest in biomechanical equipment and routines to restore and maintain one's frame. The words he contributes here are worth heeding:

Understanding the basic physics principle of applied force as it relates to structural integrity is a good first step toward understanding how you can achieve a healthy back and maintain it to keep it in top functioning shape.

When force exceeds load-bearing ability, injury must occur. Thus, as the inherent forces of nature cannot be altered in most cases, we must concern ourselves instead with enhancing the structural integrity of the lower back frame members—five lumbar vertebrae and the soft tissue that supports them: disks, cartilage, ligaments, and muscles.

You don't have to know every intricacy of back anatomy, but you should be familiar enough with the basics. Let's start with the backbone, or, more accurately, the back "bones," or vertebrae. A healthy spine forms a couple of gentle S-curves. There are built-in shock and friction absorbers and stabilizers for the two facet joints that each vertebra has with the one above it. Spongy disks, together with soft cartilage, prevent bones from directly rubbing against each other, while ligaments keep the vertebrae aligned.

You were born with a critical anatomical component that is the first line of defense against back dysfunction—deep muscles that help keep vertebrae in line, and superficial muscles that extend from the vertebrae to the ribs. It could be argued with confidence that the lower back is the most vulnerable area of the body and that the role of its muscles cannot be overstated. And that brings us to the purpose of this book.

BALANCING ACT

Your "backbone" is a protective enclave for your spinal cord, a critical anatomical part for movement. That bony architecture protects a vast network of spinal nerves: The cord runs right down the center (it's a high-speed—not a dial-up—line that transmits signals), and there are tributaries on each side that end in nerve roots in soft tissue. Your ability to sense touch in one part of your arm or leg is attributed to one nerve or another, and each muscle group is fired by a certain nerve. When it comes to back problems, they often are not related to the muscles themselves (although that's where you feel it); you are most likely having "referred pain" that comes from:

■ A herniated disk that squeezes out from where it should be—between two vertebrae— into the spinal canal or into the foramen (where the nerve exits at each level)

■ A spur or arthritis in a facet joint

Both conditions press upon or irritate nerves. While they usually have the most serious consequences, including surgery, a lot has to happen before that point, and a lot can be done before or after such conditions present to reverse course.

Muscles support the skeleton and move the body in the case of lower back muscles with flexion (lengthening of the deep and superficial muscles and contraction of the abdominals) and extension (lengthening of the abdominal muscles and contraction of the erector spinae and the gluteus maximus). Trunk rotation is produced by the external obliques and the internal obliques. Lateral flexion is primarily the responsibility of the quadratus lumborum muscle that works with the obliques, the latissimus dorsi, the iliopsoas, and the rectus abdominis on the side of the direction of movement. But enough with the anatomy lesson; what's most important is the overall message: There's a lot going on that's connected to the part of your back that hurts, and the muscles are key players.

Your lower back muscles hold your frame in place and expand and contract to accommodate all of the twists and turns of normal and athletic movement. And there's more to them than one might think at first because they

BACKBOARD

don't just work in the rear. Their sinews spread to the sides, to the front, and down your legs; a lot of what goes on biomechanically in those areas is directly connected to the spot you reach for when you have a backache.

The core of your frame is much like that of a dwelling you build, with "walls" that support the overall structure and bear measured loads. You have abdominal muscles in the front (anterior muscles), back extenders, oblique muscles, and then deep within you have the interpelvic muscles. If one wall in your house isn't in great shape, the entire structure is susceptible to collapse. And so it is with your biomechanical frame. It is a never-ending balancing act.

A strong lower back muscle network protects against the impact forces prevalent in sports, accidents, and many if not most activities of daily living. Keep your muscles toned,

primed for action, and the rest of your back members will move freely as they were designed to do, and they won't place undue stress on nerves or another lower back member, or encroach on your spinal cord. That's the key to fluid motion and the avoidance of sciatica, inflammation, tightness, and sprains. That's the key to being active and pain free.

WEAK LINKS AND STEALTH AILMENTS

Even if you're proactive regarding your fitness, weak links and stealth ailments lurk, and they're responsible for most back injuries and pain. Knowing a lot about them is far more important than anatomical knowledge because you can do something about most of them and hedge your bets against compromised movement or disability, and pain.

WEAK LINKS

"You're only as strong as your weakest link" may often be said, but that doesn't mean it doesn't always have meaning. If you're not on a comprehensive exercise regimen, whatever weak link you have will snap a lot sooner:

■ POOR AEROBIC CONDITION

Muscles need oxygen like engines need gas, and they and other frame members, such as intravertebral disks and ligaments, need blood supply to stay healthy. (Much more on the critical importance of aerobic conditioning in Step 4.)

■ OVERWEIGHT

It stands to reason that the more your frame has to support, the harder it has to work and the more susceptible to injury it is. (Step 4 also has some juicy tidbits on frame-appropriate nutrition.)

■ IMBALANCES

We touched on this in the preface, and it's something that crops up throughout these pages because of how they work against you—not only physically but also nutritionally and emotionally.

■ OLD INJURIES

This is a big one—the number-one predictor of future back ailments. Your body is just like paper, metal, and wood: Its cracks and tears and breaks can be "glued," "taped," "stapled," or "welded," but it may never be as strong as it was originally.

■ REINJURY

If I had a dime for every patient who showed up in my office with a reinjury (lower back or otherwise), there wouldn't have to be a cover price on this book. I'm not just talking about sprains; I'm talking about tears and fractures. There are a few primary reasons for this:

■ Incomplete rehabilitation

■ Strenuous recreation too soon

■ Improper warmup of affected area

■ Poor nutritional support

■ Medication camouflage

A vicious slide ensues as each rehab from injury only restores you so far, and you're not where you were before. That's your new baseline.

I won't mind it at all if no one shows up in my office for the above. That'll happen when a lot more people are on the FrameWork Lower Back Program.

■ AGING EFFECTS

Gray hairs and wrinkled skin aren't the only consequences of advancing years. There are tissue changes (cellular, biochemical, biomechanical) all over, with marked impact on your frame:

■ Probability of injury increases.

- Severity of injury increases.

- Time to heal increases.

- Degree of healing decreases.

Here's the bad news when you pass 40 years of age:

- Bone loss occurs.

- Loss of human growth hormone (HGH) and muscle mass is significant, and becomes precipitous after age 50.

- Loss of collagen and change in its structural integrity are steady (tendons and ligaments have loads of collagen).

Here's the good news: The advance of all of the above is slowed, and at times even halted or reversed, by the FrameWork Lower Back Program.

■ STRUCTURAL DEFECTS

Sometimes bridges come tumbling down. Usually, that's a consequence of wear and tear; in a few cases, it's because of an inherent design defect. Some of us have scoliosis or another vertebral anomaly—bones misshaped or "misconnected" in some way. This is one of the two lower back weak links no one can do much about.

BACKBOARD

Lesson: Weak Links

Poor Aerobic Condition

Overweight

Imbalances

Old Injuries

Reinjury

Aging Effects

Structural Defects

Genetics

■ GENETICS

The other one. It no doubt plays a role in structural defects and degenerative disk disease, but it has also been linked to arthritis and heart disease, as well as to other factors that impact the lower back: height, weight, athleticism, and . . . pain.

Yes, you read that right. A recent study by David H. Kim, MD, at Tufts University School of Medicine shed some light on why one person with a degenerated disk reports "discomfort" while another with the exact same condition clamors for serious meds. He and his team isolated two pain-modulating genes and their work points to as many as 12 others that might predict how surgical candidates respond to disk procedures. As I said, we can't do much about certain weak links, but "pains-taking" advances such as this will improve the 75 percent success rate that is associated with disk surgery.

So there you have it—the facts about potential threats to your chain of health. You'll get a lot more up close and personal with the ones most applicable to you in Step 3.

STEALTH AILMENTS

You age in a fashion that's uniquely yours, and there are things going on that you're not aware of—yet. But you will be, sure as tomorrow follows today, because the silent wear and tear below is eventually voiced in nagging aches and injuries that compromise your active life and cause pain.

■ TIGHTNESS

Most of us spend huge chunks of our day in sedentary activities or on our feet without moving about much. Cashiers, drivers, administrators, salesclerks, managers . . . the list goes on and on. Their backs are essentially put in storage, until they're asked to do some serious work, lifting or recreating, and then it's watch out—just like that, something snaps.

Those who have more active life-styles, such as nurses, firefighters, delivery people, and fitness enthusiasts, aren't necessarily out of the woods when it comes to lower back tightness. As noted above, physical imbalances can exist—even athletic, fit individuals can have imbalances from their own fitness or sports routines—and, as we'll discuss in Step 4, hardly anyone stretches properly for any activity, work or play.

■ WEAKNESS

Lower back muscle weakness is very common, and this is especially true of the lumbar extensor muscles. They are the double support system running parallel on each side of the vertebrae that you can feel in the center of your spine. They're also the muscles that feel great to get massaged when your lower back is sore. They can get quite nasty when they go into spasm, twisting you out of shape like a pretzel. Individuals who have recurrent lower back pain have been shown to have significant predictable weakness and atrophy of this important muscle group.

With other injured body parts, once you are feeling better and using the body part normally, strength and mobility return (think of a limb that was in a cast: remove the cast and there is lots of muscle loss; start using the limb and things usually revert over time to normal). This is not so for the lower back extensor muscles, which remain in a weakened dysfunctional state until awakened or rebooted with the proper exercise sequences. Until the atrophy is reversed, the spine remains very vulnerable to persistent pain and recurrent injury.

The other interesting thing about this pretty unique muscle group is that in addition to being the cornerstone of a healthy, durable lower back, once strengthened these muscles don't require as much work (i.e., exercise sessions) as most other muscle groups in

BACKBOARD

Lesson: A Healthy Lumbar Spine

The spine gets vulnerable with age, whether you're having symptoms or not, so your disks become more like raisins. Instead of being white and football-shaped, they've shriveled up and gotten darker, because they've lost some water content. And that's what happens, too, when someone injures his or her back, as I and millions of others have. The result is a more vulnerable structure with less-than-optimal shock absorption capability.

your body. A little work done right goes a long, long way.

■ **DISK DEGENERATION AND HERNIATION**
On certain MRI scan sequences, any body part with fluid in it normally comes out white, and those spongy disks of which we spoke earlier, seen from the side, appear as smoky little footballs. A disk is like a grape, filled with water and healthy, when you're young. Thirty to 40 percent of us will

BACK STORY

One of the most troubling things I see is soft bone, especially when I operate on young female athletes to reconstruct their injured knees. To replace torn ligaments through the arthroscope, I must create anchoring tunnels in the bones. To drill into the bone of an 18-year-old male, I have to use power tools and all my strength. But with too many of the young women, I can simply rotate the drill bit with my fingers and the metal will easily pass through the bone as if it were butter. You don't need to be a psychic to know they are heading for trouble.

have, by age 40, compressed, bulging disks or degenerated disks without necessarily showing any symptoms (a topic in Step 2). A study using MRI analysis was done with asymptomatic 40-year-olds who had never had a problem with their backs. Forty percent of them showed disk herniations and/or degeneration—accidents waiting to happen. On an MRI, their disks looked more like raisins than grapes, having lost most of their fluid cushion. Also, your spine can age prematurely. This can be due to genetic factors or trauma. Even repetitive overload can cause degeneration as seen in football players, power lifters, and gymnasts. Spine MRIs of college football players (before they even join the professional ranks) have shown high levels of disk degeneration and vertebral problems.

■ BONE DEGENERATION

It's no secret that elderly folks have a lot less skeletal matter than they used to in their younger days (after all, that's why they "shrink" right before our eyes), but you don't have to be very old to have significant bone loss. Osteopenia, the stage before osteoporosis, is showing up on more and more body composition scans of 50-year-olds, and the battle has been joined to stop—and even restore in some cases—bone degeneration. And the weapons aren't just new prescription drugs; they include bio-identical hormone replacement, nutrition, supplements, and . . . exercise. (Studies show that weight-bearing activity builds both muscle and bone.)

BACK STROKES

Few exercise programs address back fitness enough, so the exercise routines in Step 5 are the primary component of your FrameWork Lower Back Program. But when it comes to a comprehensive plan for back health, they're far from alone. Thus, you've got five other steps to take. Of course, you're just about finished with this one. The only thing that remains before you move on to Step 2 is a set of prescriptions for everyday living that will help you keep an active back.

▨ POSTURE

This is important enough that it's part of your self-test in Step 3. Loss of an erect frame is insidious in that decline is imperceptible as it progresses. Each incremental bend or slouch doesn't show up on our radar, but we get the (startling) picture one day when we catch ourselves in a mirror and the image doesn't jibe with the one we have in our memory.

All of us no doubt had someone in

our past who barked: "Sit up straight." For me, it was my mother. Whoever it was, the intention was to instill discipline because that's good for me and you. Form is, indeed, function in this case: An aligned frame is ideal for movement and load bearing, fatigues less easily, and is less susceptible to strain. It's an essential part of being healthy—and staying that way.

Perfect form means the heels, knees, pelvis, neck, and head are directly aligned with each other. Be sure to do your Posture Assessment assignment (above); if slippage is noticeable, make a conscious effort throughout your day to "sit up straight." It's just a matter of keeping your head erect and your shoulders "back," whether you're seated or strolling, and doing some shoulder rolls a couple of times a day to retrain your frame. (Stand with your palms next to your thighs or while holding a 5-pound weight in each hand. Rotate your upper arms and shoulders in a slow circle—backward, down, forward, and up—10 times. Repeat the set 2 more times.)

DE-STRESS YOUR SPINE

You might think sitting is restful for your back, but it can be more stressful than walking with proper posture or even heavy weight lifting in the gym.

Studies have shown that sitting for extended periods is extremely stressful on your lumbar spine. Office workers aren't the only ones at risk. People who don't sit right in the car, at the dinner table, on an airplane, or wherever else they happen to be, put tremendous stress on their lower back disks. It's no

A TIP FOR AN ACTIVE LIFE

Many of my patients swear by the newer memory-foam mattresses.

wonder that so many backs go out after long trips. Are you one of those who lies down on the floor (or even sleeps there!) to recover?

Fortunately, there are far-less-drastic measures available to keep your back "chill." Anytime you've been sitting for an hour, get up to give your disks a break, because they are maximally loaded in the seated position. And keep these other tips in the back of your mind to take a load off.

■ SIT BACK

Lengthening your spine and decompressing your disks a couple of times a day prevents damage and allows

damage to heal better. Try this simple routine; you'll like it.

Use headrests whenever possible, rest your feet on the floor (swaying feet pull on the pelvis and distort the natural curve of the back), adjust your computer monitor to eye level, and keep your elbows in line with your keyboard to minimize strain on neck and shoulder muscles.

■ SUPPORT YOUR LOCAL LUMBAR

By all means, when given the option, choose one of the many office and lounge chairs that have built-in lumbar support.

A TIP FOR AN ACTIVE LIFE

Upon awakening, stretch your neck, shoulders, arms, and legs, moving them gently in multiple directions. The safest way to rise, especially if you have back problems, is to roll to your side, assuming a fetal position and pointing your knees off the side of the bed, and as you slide your feet and legs off the side of the bed, help yourself up and off with your lower elbow and forearm.

EVERYDAY TIPS FOR AN ACTIVE LIFE

■ Take a bicycle instead of the car to work or on errands to town.

■ Park your car far from entrances.

■ Walk up and down stairways for those one or two floors to ground level, or get off the elevator two floors below where you're headed.

■ Answer phone calls standing up.

■ If you rest, you rust. So keep moving.

Auto seat design has also come a long way since I drove around in my 280Z. If you can't decide between two car models, going with the one that comfortably supports your lower back when you sit in it wouldn't be a bad way to go. When you travel by air and are imprisoned in a much-less-than-ideal chair, be sure to tuck one of those small pillows (if one is to be had) in the small of your back.

■ WATCH THOSE BLTs

This is for all those who've said or are going to say, "I just bent over the sink while brushing my teeth, and my back went out." It's about avoiding the pitfalls of bending, lifting, and twisting—the BLTs. I'm not referring to a sandwich here (although that should be avoided, too, despite its temptation); what I have in mind is how an awful lot of people use their backs like a crane, and they're not meant to be used that way. You can get in more trouble picking up a feather off the floor than you can trying to pick up a 100-pound barbell. For that, you'd likely stand square to it, bend your knees, grasp it tightly, and then rise slow and easy. But if you're in your house and there's something on the floor, you'd be of a mind to rapidly bend and twist, amplifying the stresses on the disks and facet joints.

■ PUT YOUR BACK CARES TO BED

A significant amount of lower back

BACK STORY

You can rebuild muscle at *any* age. Studies involving movement-challenged 90-year-olds showed that after a 12-week strength-building program, strength improved dramatically, as did functional capability: Those who had used walkers were able to get around with canes, and those who had used canes walked without them!

discomfort can be prevented with the right mattress. This is especially true for people who wake up with discomfort and morning stiffness in the spine. Go with one of the three or four best-selling manufacturers; I like a mattress that is slightly firm but accommodating, with a cushioned pillow-top, rather than a rigid plank design.

■ RISE AND SHINE

One of gravity's effects is that you lose height during the day, and that's partly because fluid is forced out of your disks. The disks rehydrate with nutrient-filled fluid during your sleeping hours, but the trade-off for that is that your back is most vulnerable when you wake up, because disks are plump and full again. This is why many individuals suffer "back attacks"

in the morning, even with relatively minor activities such as leaning over the sink to brush their teeth, tying their shoes, or even sitting up in bed.

A disk is somewhat like a water balloon—if it's half-filled, it doesn't burst easily; if it's filled to the brim, it doesn't take much for it to pop. We hear over and over people who say, "I was fine, I woke up, I bent over to brush my teeth or went to put some hosiery on, and boom!—I was on the floor in severe pain." A lot of people just bolt upright when they wake up, or go from lying down to standing on the floor in a heartbeat. Such sudden movements put intense pressure on your disks and muscles and connective tissue, and increase the likelihood that something will pop. Instead, when your eyes open in the morning, try the active life tip on the bottom of page 11.

And, if you're suffering with back pain, I don't recommend going right to the gym in the morning before work, as many people do. Early morning (or whenever you wake up) vulnerability can last about an hour or so. For this reason, you should be very careful with early morning workouts, or consider hitting the gym a little later in the day if your schedule permits. If you don't have another option for working out, you've got to spend extra time getting warmed up, working your problem area, rather than going into that first lift.

■ **BACK YOURSELF UP IN GENERAL**

Taking care of your back doesn't always involve a structured routine in a time period carved out specifically for it. Much good can come from your everyday lifestyle, and once you've made the couple of suggestions below part of how you move about daily, you will have acquired a habit that keeps your back active.

BACK TO BEING ACTIVE

Aging and injury and repetitive stress prey upon the components of your spine. These forces wear away cartilage, distort disks, and overstretch ligaments so they lose their elasticity (just as old rubber bands do), leading to an unstable spine. The common denominator for all lower back components is the muscle group that connects all of them, supports all of them, and controls movement of all of them.

Spinal strength is the ultimate key to spinal stability. Strengthening the musculature of the lower back is prophylactic—it will go a long way toward protecting the intricate involved anatomy. And rehabilitation of the lower back in most clinical cases depends in large measure on the strength of the involved soft tissues. And that brings us again to our purpose here—exercising your back. My good friend Roger Schwab perhaps said it best:

In changing times, trendy catchwords often spring up in everyday vocabulary. One of the more recent ones is the "core" of the body, but, in contrast to the more comprehensive FrameWork philosophy, the way it is used most of the time is in reference to the abdominal structure. The concept espouses that strengthening the abdominal muscles will go a long way to preventing and/or rehabilitating lower back injuries. Conclusive clinical experience has shown that this conclusion is in error. Abs are important, but far more integral to the functional/ structural integrity of the lower back is the development of the muscles that extend the lower back (lumbar extensors) and the muscles that rotate the torso. In other words, the lumbar extensors get individual attention in the FrameWork Lower Back Program.

Though a safe, specific-exercise paradigm is paramount for a healthy lower back, a poorly designed or random-exercise program is the antithesis of that, and it can (and too often does) create either acute or chronic problems. Many "mainstream" physical routines and recreational activities that are practiced widely are questionable. Over the years, I have seen more than a couple of well-intentioned fitness programs cause significant damage. So-called "explosive" exercise under load (against resistance) and quick, sudden stop-and-start exercises can compromise structural integrity. Although an acute injury will present itself almost immediately (and painfully), many orthopaedic problems

will not be immediately apparent; rather, bodily stress accumulates gradually, resulting in breakdown, dysfunction, and pain after a period of time.

This is often the issue in lower back cases. Constant force on the non-shored-up lumbar spine, on the atrophied surrounding soft tissues, will result in pain there over time. If the safe, targeted FrameWork protocols herein are put into action, the frequency, intensity, and duration of lower back pain will be drastically reduced. Of equal importance, if intense, isolated exercise is used as a prerequisite for intense physical activity or recreational sport, participants will prevent the pulls and tears that have long plagued men and women of all ages.

Let me repeat: Sedentary is not an option. And regular golf or tennis or aerobics or circuit training isn't enough either. If you want to stay healthy or recover faster and more completely from back injury and pain, there's no choice but to build up muscle and functional capability with the comprehensive cross-training and support recommendations in these pages.

It's time to take the next step.

Your Out-of-Whack Back

This part of the journey to lower back health isn't just for the millions who are suffering or hobbled in some way right now because of a back ailment. It's a cautionary tale for anyone who wants to avoid back problems or recover from one that visits down the road.

The tale is in the numbers, but I won't overwhelm you with math here; it'll suffice just to give you the National Center for Health Statistics "background" data from 2004 on the massive financial and social impact of lower back incidences and treatment.

- Twelve to 15 percent of the US population showed up in a doctor's office and reported lower back pain. It was the leading primary-care complaint, more than 44 million times.

- Forty-three to 60 percent of adults reported experiencing neck or lower back pain in the previous 3 months.

- Lower back pain prevalence increases with age.

- Overall, almost one out of every two people experiences back pain at least once a year.

- A reported 33.7 million people spent one or more days in bed in the previous year because of back pain.

- Although 90 percent of patients suffering from their first episode of back pain will be asymptomatic within 3 months, 40 to 60 percent will predictably have recurrent episodes.

- Estimated annual direct medical costs for all spine-related conditions were $193.9 billion (an average of almost $6,000 for each patient), and back pain was responsible for $30.3 billion of that amount. The total represents 5 percent of all health-care visits to physicians, clinics, and hospitals.

- Annual indirect cost in lost wages as a result of spine disorders was $14 billion.

The hard facts above only confirm what pretty much everyone knows from personal experience. If you happen to be that rare individual who's never had a back ailment and doesn't know someone who has had one, you wouldn't have to go very far or search very hard to find such a person. Sooner or later, one of these back complaints will make itself known to just about everyone.

■ MUSCLE SPRAINS AND STRAINS

As I said earlier, muscle "pulls" are almost exclusively reserved for young adults who play as hard as they work and demand more from their bodies than what they were designed to do. They don't accept limitations and are unacquainted with the concept of mortality, so they sometimes stretch their muscles to the point of injury. Youth being what it is, a little ice and/ or heat and/or an elastic wrap, and they're good to go in no time.

You are as young as your spine, say the yoga masters.

For the rest of us older folks, pulls happen off the court as much as on it; they occur after sudden movements or as a result of seemingly innocuous bends and turns. The so-called pulls are usually a deeper issue, with the muscle pain being a secondary response—the muscle ache is the smoke alarm, and the fire is somewhere else to be found. There are causes other than athletic exuberance, deeper malfunctions behind these strains, that can be traced to other frame members—first and foremost to those spongy "grapes" that cushion vertebrae.

■ DISK WOES

Disk degeneration is a natural result of aging, but in most cases there aren't any symptoms related to it for quite some time. Sometimes, disk degeneration can occur earlier in life if you have experienced an injury, if you have repeated exposure to certain sports, or even if you just happen to have the wrong genetic makeup. Yes, blame your parents or ancestors in some cases. Your disks will do what they do—lose fluid, compress, and not rebound all the way, encroaching on adjacent territory— and you will do what you do—go about your day-to-day life, none the wiser about what is going on with your frame.

Until the silence is broken.

Loudly.

By shooting pain.

And severe restriction of movement.

Your back cries out when disk degeneration, or associated spurs, has progressed to the point where a disk presses on a nerve. Your pain can also radiate into your buttock or leg.

Another common problem with disks is that they can move out of place. Instead of the disk staying centered between the vertebrae, the disk's material slips out toward the spinal canal. It can move left, right, center, or all of the above. What starts out as a bulge can then become a full-blown herniation. These herniations are very common and are often without any symptoms whatsoever. However, in its new resting place, a herniated disk can also cause major problems. It can press on nerves coming from the spinal cord and exiting the spinal area through the foramina (the small passageways through which nerves travel from the

BACK STORY

I'm always concerned about keeping up with my patient visit schedule because I'm hypersensitive about the fact that nobody likes to wait to be seen, especially busy executives and other people with tight schedules who take up a large chunk of my calendar. But I never know what's behind the next door and can't predict how long any given patient will take, so slippage is unavoidable.

When I first went into practice, I'd get a feel for whether I was keeping up with appointments by observing how crowded the waiting room was. Out of the corner of my eye, I'd see people pacing back and forth and think, "Oh no, they're *really* impatient—and probably upset with me, too." I'd really fret when I saw patients who had been waiting for me in an exam room pacing back and forth in that confined space—until it finally dawned on me that sitting was very uncomfortable for people who had sciatica and other back problems. Figuratively slapping my forehead with the palm of my hand, I realized these patients of mine weren't antsy—their backs were "out of whack"!

spinal cord out past the spinal canal). When the nerve gets crunched, the result can range from a little numbness or radiating pain in the buttocks or legs to full-blown weakness in certain muscles in the leg or foot. The leg pain associated with a disk herniation is called sciatica. Much more rarely, there can be major pressure on the spinal cord resulting in significant leg weakness and even bowel or bladder dysfunction. This so-called cauda equina syndrome, an absolute "red flag," is a true medical and surgical emergency, one of the few lower back problems that require prompt surgical intervention. (More red flags below.)

Disk degeneration is the genesis of misalignment of other frame members that leads to additional common lower back complaints.

▪ ARTHRITIS

When disks bulge, vertebrae get closer to each other and abnormal movement occurs, wearing away the thin layer of cartilage that covers your back bones. Over time, inflammation develops that irritates nerves nearby. Like arthritis anywhere else in your body, spinal arthritis can be a source of significant symptoms, pain, and limitation of activity.

▪ FACET JOINT SYNDROME

Ongoing friction causes spurs to form where vertebrae are closest to each other—the facet joints. Without intervention, spurs continue to grow until they, too, invade the foramina. When facet joints fail, abnormal movement and even instability result. A bad facet joint can cause buttock or thigh pain that can be confused with the more traditional sciatica related to disk herniations.

▪ SPINAL STENOSIS

Left unchecked, disk degeneration, arthritis, and spurs conspire to narrow the spinal canal within your vertebrae. The eventual consequence is constant pressure on nerves at one or multiple levels, resulting in significant pain that shoots down the legs.

These pinched nerves can also cause neurogenic claudication—progressive pain when walking—that is similar to the vascular claudication experienced by those who have arterial or blood vessel disease in the legs. Nerves in the legs weaken more and more from constant compression and "go dead" at times, necessitating frequent stops when you take a stroll.

◼ SACROILIAC (SI) JOINT DYSFUNCTION

Your spine attaches to the two sides of your pelvis via SI joints. For years, doctors thought that SI joints couldn't "sublux" (go out on you) and be a real cause of discomfort or pain, but it's generally accepted now by spine experts that these joints can be problematic, another consequence of frame member malfunction.

Not all buttock or leg pain is caused by a pinched nerve. If your sacroiliac joint is out of alignment, it can get irritated and inflamed, and that can lead to radiating pain.

BACK STORY

Ever since I injured my back horsing around on the beach, SI joint dysfunction has certainly been an issue for me. It goes out pretty easily. I'll get twisted like a pretzel, my spine will lock up, and I'll be in a lot of discomfort. Dr. Neil Liebman, a really terrific chiropractor, refers to this condition as the "safety pin cycle," meaning the body is unable to correct it on its own.

It's sometimes hard to get it right, especially when I'm really hurting. Basically, Neil has one shot at it, but he has tremendous hands and gets things back in place and the muscles out of spasm. "It's almost like reading Braille," he says. "The correction of these misalignments is gentle, very safe, and requires little force with the new technology that is available."

I give Neil a lot of credit for getting me over humps—I don't think exercise alone would have worked as well. A lot of doctors pooh-pooh the subluxations that chiropractors talk about. Call it what you will, they are definitely moving things around, and that often provides immediate relief if you're locked into a situation where an SI or facet joint is bothering you. Then it is up to you to do the proper preventive or curative exercise routines. You cannot just rely on manipulation all the time; it provides the "quick fix," but proper exercise offers the long-term solution.

Most of the time, lower back ailments have a recurrent nature: They come, stay a while, and go away until next time. They can show up during or after prolonged activity, or for a reason that defies reasonable explanation. For some, chronic back pain is an almost-constant companion. Whatever the case is, these ailments are something we're used to dealing with and can get past after the usual inconvenience and discomfort.

Then there's the other kind of back problem: a sudden "pop" that elicits an "Oh, no!" Pain aside, it's quite worrisome in that it's unlike anything else you've experienced, brought on by bending, sudden movement, or an extra-strenuous load on your frame. The exact source of these acute episodes cannot usually be pinned down. Sometimes, they can be traced to:

■ An annular tear: The annulus fibrosus ligament that wraps a disk can split or separate from it.

■ A compression fracture: Osteoporosis—usually in older people—weakens verte-brae that "crack" under pressure. (I have even seen this in elderly women who tried to open a stuck window.)

■ Acute disk herniation: "Pop" goes the disk, and down you go.

■ Muscle or ligament strains.

IS IT INJURY . . . OR "JUST" PAIN?

Here's the short recap: Millions of people are affected by one or more lower back ailments. Here's what comes next: The pain associated with those ailments is deceptive.

It frightens you, yes, and tells your body not to do things, but it turns out that most of the time we overreact to its message as we do when that oversensitive smoke alarm goes off and brings the fire department to our homes, and all we were doing was making toast or lighting a few birthday candles. So how do we overre-spond in terms of our back attacks? By crawl-ing into bed for more than a day or two, by taking serious and potentially dangerous drugs, by severely restricting activity, and by seeking "magic bullets"—the more drastic trac-tion and surgery. Fear and impatience can sure take you down some seriously wrong paths.

It is critically important to understand the difference between *hurt* and *harm*. This is something we sports team physicians deal with all the time when we work with professional athletes and have to decide if they can go back in and compete with certain ailments or injuries. Some just hurt, and further activity will not harm things. For others we insist that they remain sidelined because going back into battle could make the situation worse with immediate or long-term harm. "It may hurt a little" or "it will harm you"—worlds of difference between the two.

Many lower back problems are so uncomfortable or painful that you get frightened and wrongly assume that movement and activity will harm you. Nothing can be further from the truth. Rarely, conditions necessitate severe activity restriction; usually, modified appropriate activities, sooner rather than later, are called for.

You should talk to your doctor or healthcare provider to get some clarification as to where you stand—and hopefully get reassurance as well as a license to move. I recently saw a US Marine T-shirt with the statement PAIN IS WEAKNESS LEAVING THE BODY. Although I can't fully subscribe to that in all instances, I do believe there is some truth in it. Sometimes you do need to work through some nonharmful discomfort to get out of a bad situation.

Admittedly, "disk degeneration" and "disk herniation" sound alarming, and both conditions look ominous on a light box in your doctor's office, but there's a real upside for patients in those diagnoses (aside from having an explanation for persistent pain). You see, several studies using serial MRIs have shown gradual reabsorption and even disappearance of herniated disks—including some large ones— in some cases. Further research into how this occurs showed that your body actually creates an enzyme to repair those shock absorbers between your vertebrae. Even if your disk does not reabsorb and disappear spontaneously, you can still be fine. In fact, most patients with confirmed, painful herniated disks recover *without surgery* in 1 to 6 months!

Back pain resolves spontaneously in most patients.

And there's similar good news for those whose lower back pain is idiopathic (with an unknown cause): The American Academy of Orthopaedic Surgeons says that "back pain resolves spontaneously in most patients." This includes acute cases that can heal in as little as 2 weeks, and sciatica—even some of the cases that involve numbness and/or weakness—although it might take 12 or more weeks to clear up.

So it seems that the centuries-old dictum to medical students, *Primum non nocere* (First, do no harm), is quite appropriate for back complaints. But it doesn't apply just to doctors—a back patient must be "patient" as well. This doesn't mean, however, that *nothing* should be done. Far from it.

Pain can lead to disuse, which leads to atrophy, which can lead to true disability. We may not have a choice about being inactive with some conditions, such as bone fractures that require casts, but that doesn't apply to the majority of back ailments. Research has radically changed the way we approach back pain (that's the second half of this step), and here's the skinny once again: Being sedentary is not an option. Remember, "motion is lotion."

Pain can lead to disuse, which leads to atrophy, which can lead to true disability.

My colleague and friend Vert Mooney, MD, was a renowned San Diego spine expert and surgeon who gave up doing surgeries to focus on rehabilitation of lower back conditions. Perhaps this is because he and other research-

ers have demonstrated that progressive lumbar strength training has significant potential to reduce the need for spine operations. He is a visionary with a wealth of experience, and he shares his thoughts on pain, its management, and how to reverse it:

Patients tend to look for miracles. Given the current interest in the traction devices, this is an example of how far they will go. Most of these treatment programs are not covered by any insurance, and yet folks will pay over $2,000 for intermittent traction. Of course, there has never been a scientific paper that showed that this had any long-term beneficial effect.

When the pain is acute and unrelenting and seems to follow neurologic pathways, that is worrisome. Nonetheless, that is quite a rare event. Most of the time, pain in the extremities is on a referred basis and reversible by appropriate exercise programs. As long as the pain is intermittent and can be changed by posture and activity, it is not a worrisome area of concern.

As we all know, pain can often be quite nicely abolished by chiropractic care. The downside of this is that the res-

olution of the pain by this mode does not seem to be permanent. In my experience, the only maneuver to get longer-term relief of pain is an active, progressive exercise program. This, in my mind, should include resistance exercises as well as range of motion. The bottom line from a patient standpoint is that pain is certainly a point of concern, but it is usually just a warning and not something to be considered a permanent problem.

Of course, in situations where anatomy has gone awry, such as in spinal stenosis with progressive pain [that accompanies] physical activity and herniated disks with neurologic deficits, surgical care is often the ideal solution. There is significant indication that this solution is more effective the sooner the better.

The reason back surgery has such a bad reputation is that a lot of people feel that they're pushed into a corner. They keep going back to their doctors' offices with the same complaint of severe pain, then frustration sets in for both the patient and physician, and too often doctors throw their hands up and say, "Let's operate." But in many cases they're not operating for the right reasons. If you have a significantly pinched nerve or weakness down the leg, and conservative measures have failed, that's where back surgery can be very, very successful, and it's appropriate in a couple of other instances outlined a little later. But if you're trying to use surgery to cure a common backache that, as we've mentioned, could be associated with one or more frame members, the prognosis isn't very promising at all. Believe it or not, back surgery is usually more appropriate for leg-related symptoms (i.e., sciatica, weakness, or claudication) than for backache alone.

Spine surgery is not a cure-all for back pain.

Migraine headaches can be very incapacitating, but we don't do brain surgery to cure them, even if the patient suffers daily with them. The severity of symptoms should never be a trigger to make a wrong decision, especially when it comes to surgery. In that regard, backache and back pain can be viewed like a migraine headache, where surgery is not a magic bullet.

Spine surgery is not a cure-all for back pain. I know, when you're in agony it can be mighty hard to trust that the pain will go away on its own, but the odds are overwhelmingly in your

BACK STORY

favor if you don't have a specific indication for surgical intervention. You must be very care-ful and not go down the surgery path too quickly. If you and your doctor are thinking surgery, you should get another opinion from another medical professional who has a great reputation and is honest. And you should be aware of regional influences on the preva-lence of particular surgeries.

There were studies done at Dartmouth Medical School and other institutions on the geographical variation in surgical procedures that should serve as a warning for anyone con-sidering a back operation. Why is it that in Philadelphia, for example, you're more likely to have surgery for a sore knee than in some other major cities? Why is lumbar fusion surgery performed 20 times more often in Idaho Falls than in Bangor, Maine? Why is the likelihood of having back surgery directly related to the number of fellowship-trained spine surgeons in a given area? It has to do with the training and the philosophy that is prominent in the locale. As has been said, when all you have is a hammer, everything looks like a nail. So some doctors are more apt to suggest or perform sur-gery than others.

In reality, and ideally, the decision about when to operate and when not to, and on whom, should not vary widely from town to town. Some may be operating too much and others too little. Either way, geographic variation is something we in the medical profession need to better understand and explain, and it is some-thing you as a patient need to be aware of.

Some doctors are more apt to suggest or perform surgery than others.

For some people, however, surgery is the right answer up front. And as Dr. Mooney advises, the sooner the better in certain spe-cific instances. But for most of the typical lower back conditions, surgery is not warranted at all because the ailments get better on their own (and faster with the self-help recommendations below). You might feel better in the near term with surgery if you have a herniated disk with significant sciatica; if you take the pressure off that nerve, you might feel better sooner and get back to work quicker, which is a good enough reason for some people to do it. But studies show that 5 years down the line, whether you've had surgery or not for that herniated disk, the two groups seem to do equally well. What this means is that surgery or not, 5 years later each group has the same number of patients who feel great as well as the same number with ongoing lower back complaints.

So you have to be careful about surgery and resist the thinking that you just want to "get this over with," unless it's an absolute emergency where you're going downhill quickly. You need somebody to really help you make the right decision. You must go to a highly regarded spine surgeon who doesn't have a reputation for being too quick to recommend surgery, and get another opinion from another reputable person. (It might seem crazy to some people that a surgeon like me is telling you that you have to be careful when you go

BACK STORY

When patients show up in my office with both back and leg pain, I ask, "If I could snap my fingers and get rid of either the back or leg pain, which would you prefer?" They almost always say the back pain. When they say leg pain, I'd be more likely to order an MRI. Most of the time we find a couple of issues on film and aren't 100 percent sure which is the culprit, but the good news is we tackle a lot of them with the same approach. If their leg pain doesn't come around, I'll refer them to a spine specialist.

to see a surgeon, but that's the way I'm "cut.")

For the vast majority of people who have the occasional situation when their back goes out, it's like the storm that passes through or the common cold—it's going to run its course. You've got to weather it, batten down the hatches or take the cold medicines that make you feel a little better, but they don't make the storm or cold end any quicker. With back ailments, however, a couple of things will make it end sooner: being in better physical shape from the get-go, and using first aid approaches that include chiropractic, which studies have shown can get you out of an acute episode faster. Also, there are specialized nerve blocks that can be done to help the situation in some instances.

The more fit you and your back are, the less likely you are to have "back attacks." And if you do have one, it tends to be less severe and not last as long as for those who are deconditioned and out of shape.

Most of the time, we simply don't know for sure why your back hurts, what the specific trigger is. A lot of times a combination of factors is involved: On your MRI, we might see three levels where disks are beat up; one disk has a marked herniation on the right, but all of the pain is on your left; you have a couple of facet joints that are narrowing. Heck, it might even be because you have a kidney or gallbladder stone. So who knows exactly what the cause is? It's often a case where doctors are not as smart as we think we are.

"For a vast number of people," said orthopaedic surgeon Howard S. An in the November 2008 issue of *Ladies' Home Journal*, "back pain comes from multiple sources, and we're just not sure why it hurts so much." But unless you're a definitive surgical case that requires doctors to pinpoint the cause (because they don't go into your spine with a shotgun approach), it doesn't really matter. For the majority of us, back pain isn't going to be cured with back surgery.

What does matter is what you *can* do about it. But before we get to that (and there's quite a lot, actually), we have to be sure we know when there isn't any option other than going under the knife.

RED FLAGS

Although surgery is not indicated in the vast majority of cases, there are times when you should *stop* everything and see an orthopaedic surgeon or visit an ER right away.

- Leg pain and/or numbness (especially below the knee), leg weakness (claudication), or loss of muscle function (such as a "dropped foot")

- Night pain (can't sleep at all), or pain when resting

- A disk herniation that is so large it presses on an entire nerve plexus, causing bowel or bladder dysfunction

- Trauma associated with certain fractures

- Spinal instability—one or more vertebrae slip forward when the back is in a flexed or extended position

- Lumbar stenosis (nerve canal narrowing) that results in unremitting pressure on nerves and constant pain

- Tumor or infection (an abscess) that is indicated by back pain, unexplained weight loss, and/or fever

- Aneurysm in the abdominal aorta

- Cauda equina syndrome—nerve roots in the lumbar region, especially those that control bladder and bowel function, are compressed and paralyzed, cutting off sensation and movement

If there is concern for any of the above (by you, your family doctor, or any health care practitioner), then you need immediate surgical evaluation, so get thee to a spine surgeon, a hospital, or an ER!

YOUR SURGICAL CONSULTATION

When you have constant back and leg pain, especially if the leg pain is getting worse, then it's time to get an evaluation by a surgeon. When you go to see an orthopaedic surgeon or neurosurgeon, he or she will inquire about your medical history (diabetes and immuno-deficiency could explain an infection) and ask about leg symptoms. The physical examination will include gait evaluation, hip exam, spinal flexibility assessment, motor strength testing (hip to toes), and assessment of reflexes. You'll walk on your tiptoes and on your heels, and get tapped by that little hammer on your knees and ankles. You'll get your leg checked for nerve irritation with a "straight leg raise" test—the leg is brought up, almost like a hamstring stretch, putting tension on the nerve root that will reproduce sciatica if you have it. The surgeon will also ask if you smoke, and for a very good reason (Step 4 covers that in depth).

In 2004, two procedures accounted for 66 percent of all spine surgeries:

- Diskectomy (34 percent, or more than 325,000 cases): This surgery involves removing a disk to relieve pressure on a nerve root. Scar tissue fills in the vacated area in a short time. This procedure usually includes a lumbar laminectomy, in which a small amount of bone is removed to access the damaged disk and pinched nerve. When this surgery is done through smaller mini-incisions, it is called a micro-diskectomy.

- Spinal fusion (32 percent): Supplemental bone material (autografts or allografts) is used in conjunction with the body's natural osteoblastic (bone forming) processes to immobilize vertebrae that move abnormally

BACKBOARD

and cause pain. The fusion can involve multiple levels. The more levels involved, the bigger the surgery.

Other procedures can be performed, including the use of screws and connectors that stabilize the spine, and the still-evolving implantation of artificial disks (more on that later).

If the evidence for surgery isn't clear-cut, your doctor may recommend conservative measures such as physical therapy, acupuncture, or nerve blocks. Some physicians might suggest spinal decompression therapy (computer-controlled intermittent motorized or hydraulic traction), although there is not much good science to support this sophisticated and expensive traction device.

The most thorough surgical consultation will also include an evaluation of psychological factors that can be responsible for chronic pain, pain amplification, and surgery-seeking behavior, and of other psychosocial factors that can affect the outcome of surgical procedures. (There's a lot more on how your "mind frame" impacts your back health in Step 4.) Among the latest research findings are:

■ Preoperative anxiety is associated with higher levels of postoperative pain.

■ Symptoms of psychological distress may predict individual differences in pain-treatment-related outcomes (e.g., higher levels of depressive and anxious symptomatology are associated with greater pain and disability after treatment).

■ Depression is most likely to predict long-term pain and functional disability.

■ Mood, attitude, social support, coping mechanisms, and personality factors affect positive and negative surgical outcomes.

■ An optimistic outlook promotes a faster recovery and return to performing daily activities without pain.

■ When it comes to back pain, psychological distress is a more reliable predictor of the problem than MRI imaging and other sophisticated diagnostic testing.

So don't be surprised if your doctor administers the Minnesota Multiphasic Personality Inventory (MMPI) or the Distress and Risk Assessment Method (DRAM), or refers you to a psychological professional for evaluation before he or she schedules you for surgery.

As important as these psychosocial issues are, recent research has documented that far too many surgeons are not very good at identifying those patients in need of psychological evaluation and intervention. Also, for those who are indeed aware of these important issues, there's often a discomfort in dealing with it directly, and a disconnect in getting the patients the support that they need.

GET BACK TO HEALTH

Although surgical intervention is ruled out in most cases, you're still left with an aching back that nags at you and keeps you from an active lifestyle that is paramount for good health. You could wait around until someone else tells you what to do or until your episode subsides (as research proves it will sooner or later)—or you can take a proactive approach to speed things along. Even if you have had surgery, or are considering surgery, you are not off the hook in terms of the need for exercise and other preventive maintenance for your back. You probably need it more than ever.

Harry Herkowitz, MD, is a leading spine surgeon and is the director of spine surgery at the William Beaumont Hospital in Royal Oak, MI. As lead author and editor of the bible of spine care, Rothman-Simeone's *The Spine*, Herkowitz echoes the importance of spinal strength for those who have back problems, with or without surgery. According to Dr. Herkowitz, "strengthening spinal muscles is paramount in the treatment of spinal pain. Furthermore, rehabilitation of these muscles after surgical intervention may take months to years before their maximal strength is obtained."

Each case is unique; what works for someone else may not work for you, and what works for you one time may not be comfortable for the next back attack. A measure of trial and error (T & E) is called for when considering your options for getting relief and recovering from discomfort and pain. Find out what's really provocative for you, and avoid that part of the lower back treatments and workouts. Know your own body—and don't push too hard to eliminate pain and, later, to maintain your frame so you, too, won't do harm to yourself.

The key to getting "back" quickly and effectively is *movement* as soon as possible after the initial crisis is brought under control with close-at-hand self-remedies that should be used before you resort to the more extensive pain relief approaches in Step 6.

FIRST FIRST AID

Searing pain and severe restriction of mobility are managed with a combination of approaches:

■ BED REST

We now know that the old idea of staying in bed for an extended period can be harmful for your out-of-whack back because it weakens those frame members that are critical for recovery

BACK STORY

When muscles, ligaments, or tendons tear, scar tissue forms. However, studies show that appropriate, controlled movement shortly after injury causes scar tissue to form in line with the normal muscle fibers instead of forming in a haphazard way across them. The result is a healthier, more resilient type of scar tissue. So if you get going as soon as possible after a setback, your muscles and other tissues will heal better, and a reinjury will be much less likely.

and lengthens the time it takes to get you back to normal. When you are really hurting and incapacitated, a day—or, at most, two—of being off your feet is now the standard recommendation in most cases.

By all means, crawl into bed to stem the initial torment and get into the fetal or other position that is most comfortable for you. Try experimenting with pillows in strategic places (especially two or three under your knees when lying on your back) to help ease your pain. But this should only be used as an opportunity to catch your breath before embarking upon the proven course that will really solve the problem.

■ OTC MEDICATIONS

There's an entire shelf in the pharmacy of wonderful products that deliver pain relief and reduce inflammation, addressing the two things that come with every out-of-whack back.

This is a situation where T & E applies—some people respond better to ibuprofen, others get better results with acetaminophen, still others with naproxen sodium, and many rely on

BACK STORY

A woman named Yamuna Zake (www.yamunabodyrolling.com) has a terrific "body rolling" system and program that you can use to massage yourself and relieve pain. Her device is like a miniature soft basketball—I have one, and whenever my back acts up, I lie down on it and roll back and forth and side to side.

With my back, I find that my thoracic area goes out first, and that's a prelude to my SI joint and lower back going out, so before that happens I'll get on the floor and roll around a bit. I know I've prevented many minor episodes from escalating.

You could also use two tennis balls taped together, but with a finger breadth of space between them: Wrap duct tape or gorilla tape around each ball and crisscross between them; they'll fit perfectly into the paraspinal muscles on either side of the vertebral spines (the little bony bumps running down the center of your spine) and provide a deep massage.

---

plain old aspirin. (But check with your doctor before taking anything, to make sure it won't interfere with other conditions you have or drugs you are on to treat them. And follow the product's directions to the letter—prolonged use of some OTC medications can damage the liver, kidneys, or other vital organs.)

Regardless of what you choose, all of these remedies should be considered only as a short-term strategy to lessen your discomfort so you can "move" on. As for the prescription narcotics, muscle relaxers, and sedatives (part of Step 6)

that a lot of back patients ask their doctors for immediately, they don't solve the problem and are fraught with risk.

▇ TOPICAL RELIEF

Ice works wonders initially to halt acute spasms and reduce pain and inflammation. Be careful with freezer gel packs that can get as cold as your freezer and cause frostbite. Wrap them in a washcloth moistened with cool water first, then alternate for about 15 minutes on and 15 minutes off. Some individuals do better with heat,

BACKBOARD

Lesson: Second First Aid

General Movement

Massage

Chiropractic

especially the more chronic cases or those who have stiffness and/or arthritis. It helps get your blood circulating, which will speed healing and enable you to use the muscles critical for recovery.

Again, T & E will tell you how long to use each of these therapies; some people find that using one more than the other works best. Product advances in this area have been significant, and, again, there's a lot to choose from: gels, infrared heating pads, and long-lasting patches. And don't discount the benefit of warm showers, or even a hot tub. Experiment a little—and, discomfort aside, have fun!

■ RELAXATION BREATHING

Unconsciously, most of us take shallow breaths all day long; that is the rule when we are in pain (or in an excited or agitated state), and it actually produces or exacerbates stress.

The following routine is so simple that you can do it anywhere, anytime, and it's something you should do a few times every day whether or not you're experiencing pain. During acute episodes, you can do this while lying down. Once you're up and about, it can be done lying, sitting, or standing. Keep your eyes closed during all of the steps in this routine.

1. Find a quiet place and get comfortable. Try to relax and let go of tension in your body.

2. Notice your regular breathing—feel it expanding your lungs, then emptying from your lungs.

3. Take deeper breaths and notice how the infusion of additional oxygen clears your head. Focus exclusively on this, driving everything else from your mind.

4. Take even deeper breaths slowly through your nose. Hold for 1 to 2 seconds. Release the air through your mouth while relaxing your entire body. Repeat three times.

5. Breathe normally through your nose three times, focusing on the oxygen coming into your body and thinking about it expanding your chest, entering your bloodstream, and circulating from your forehead to your toes.

6. Continue taking slow, deep breaths

through your nose, but now let your belly expand so that you're breathing with your diaphragm. When your lungs are full, hold the breath for 2 seconds. (Until you get this deeper breathing down, place your palms on your abdominal area and actually feel your abdomen expand.)

7. Release the breath slowly through your mouth and exhale until your lungs feel completely empty—contract your belly to force out every last air molecule. (If your palms are still on your abdomen, you will feel it deflate and slightly tighten at the end when all of your air is exhaled.) Wait 2 seconds.

8. Repeat the cycle three times starting with Step 4 (opposite).

SECOND FIRST AID

The research is irrefutable that motion helps pain recede, speeds recovery, and ensures that the next episode (if there is one) won't have a cumulative effect that further weakens your frame.

Don't worry if you're still feeling some pain, as it's more than likely that will be the case. The sooner you get to these approaches, the better.

■ GENERAL MOVEMENT

The sole objective here is to prepare

BACKBOARD

Lesson: Third First Aid

EXTENSION

Pre-Cobra

Mid-Cobra

Cobra

FLEXION

Pelvic Tilt

Knee-to-Chest

T-Roll

your body for the transition to the approaches that follow.

Walking (gingerly) is a good thing, so get on your feet as soon as possible. Many patients find that walking in a pool is easiest to do, so try that if one is available. It's very comforting and therapeutic, is easy on the spine, and works many of the important muscles in a low-impact environment. You might find that floating with a foam noodle, or some light swimming, works even better for you.

Breaking a sweat on an elliptical machine or stationary bike is another option. Loosen things up a bit for a day or two, and stay away from those BLTs we talked about in Step 1.

BACK STORY

Because of my past injury, my back is vulnerable. It tightens up and I get into a twisted rut—the muscles don't function properly. So I get into this loss of mobility and the ability to bend in one part of the spine. And my muscles, because they're not being used properly, tighten and shorten abnormally and sometimes go into spasm. They can even atrophy, and then I get into a vicious cycle.

For the 12 years I was the doctor for the 76ers NBA team, Dr. Neil Liebman was the team chiropractor. Once the players were out on the court, we could steal some time for him to work on me, and I'd get some regular adjustments that my schedule would never otherwise allow. I had the advantage of having his wonderful hands work on me pretty frequently, and he would mobilize the affected segments and get them working so I could do the lower back workout program here that provides lasting relief.

■ MASSAGE

From personal experience and a review of the many studies that showed faster recovery from sports injuries, I'm a big believer in this approach for pain relief and locomotion support. Certified massage therapists can work wonders in terms of getting the kinks out.

You don't always have to schedule a session with a professional deep-tissue therapist—slide into a hot tub if one's available, or, better yet, recruit your significant other to rub your aches and pains away.

■ CHIROPRACTIC

As you've read, I'm a big believer in manipulation to get past a back episode or to head off one in the early stages. If you don't have a DC, find one—he or she could make all the difference between prolonged disability and a faster return to normal life.

Dr. Mike Tancredi, the chiropractor for the World Champion Philadelphia Phillies, is no stranger to keeping people going and functioning at very high levels. His recipe for spinal health is well summed up—"I feel spinal strengthening is the single most important thing a person with neck and back pain can do in order to stay out of doctors' offices. The benefits of the proper use of manipulation, passive modalities, and flexibility exercises are usually only short-lived if the patient does not get stronger and stay that way!"

THIRD FIRST AID

The approaches just discussed put you in a position to utilize the final weapon—exercise—to overcome your out-of-whack back and enable you to use the full lower back health program in Step 5. The role of exercise in the management of lower back conditions has evolved over the years. In the past, the main focus was all in the abdominal area with "flexion-based" routines such as Williams's flexion exercises. This changed when a New Zealand physiotherapist, Robin McKenzie, accidentally realized that certain static positions, especially lumbar extension, could instantly help relieve back pain.

McKenzie began to experiment with a variety of positions (repeated flexion or extension, both standing and lying) and learned that different patients respond differently, but a *majority* of patients did have one directional preference in terms of relieving their lower back symptoms. Interestingly, more patients seemed to fare better in extension than in flexion.

He developed evaluation and treatment protocols that are now used. Research has shown that disks tend to get overloaded in flexion, whereas posterior elements like facet joints are relieved with flexion. This is why folks with disk herniations usually do better in extension, and individuals with facet joint syndrome, arthritis, and spinal stenosis may prefer flexion.

I have found, with my own lower back issues, that both flexion and extension exercises and positions can be incorporated. You will need to experiment to see which *initial* exercises and movement patterns are right for you. The key is to try the flexion and extension moves that follow and note which make things feel a little better and which, if any, exacerbate or increase your symptoms. If you find one particular exercise or position that really helps, spend more time on that until your acute episode subsides. Once you are feeling better, add additional exercises.

Keep a journal of your response to these exercises and positions. Always start slowly and gently, and do not force any movements. Slight discomfort is okay, but you should not experience significant worsening of discomfort.

Extension Routines

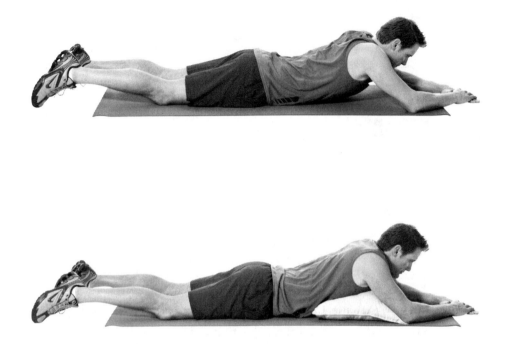

Pre-Cobra

Lie on your stomach on the floor or on a mat or with one or two pillows under your chest (which-ever is more comfortable) to create a gentle arch in your back. Hold for 2 to 3 minutes and see how you feel. If this isn't tolerable, skip to the flexion routines; if it is, repeat two times.

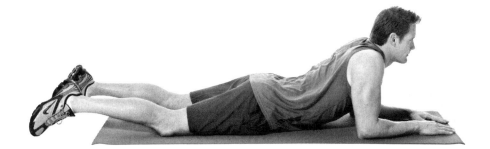

Mid-Cobra

Lie down as in the Pre-Cobra but without pillows. Raise yourself on your elbows positioned directly under your shoulders, and keep your hips and pelvis on the floor at all times. Hold for 2 to 3 minutes. Skip to the flexion routines starting on page 41 if this causes too much discomfort; otherwise, repeat two times.

Extension Routines

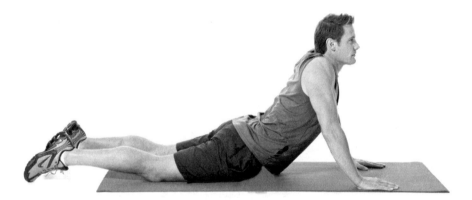

Cobra

Lie down as in the Mid-Cobra and then raise yourself, keeping your hips and pelvis on the floor, until your upper body is supported by your palms. Hold for 2 to 3 minutes. If you can do this advanced routine without excessive difficulty, repeat two times.

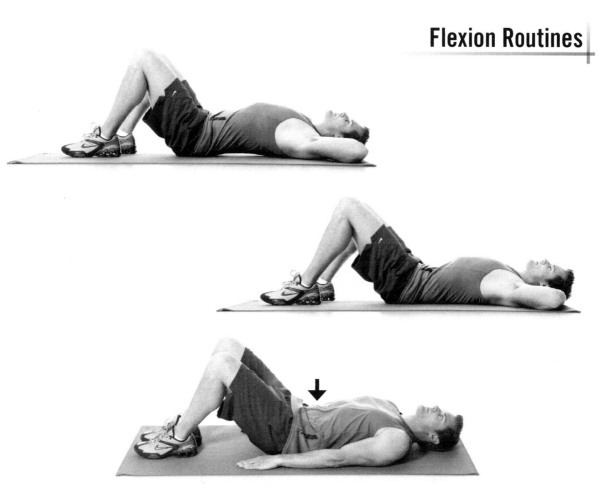

Pelvic Tilt

This routine will be the key to any exercises you do
because it teaches you to stabilize your back.

Lie on your back with your knees bent and feet flat on the floor. Pull in your stomach, bringing your belly button toward your spine, tightening your abdominal area. Also gently tighten your gluteal (buttock) muscles. Hold your abdominal area tight, concentrating on a spot approximately 2 inches below your belly button. (You should feel the small of your back flatten toward the floor, reversing the normal curve or arch of your back—but don't try to overflatten your back.) Hold this position for 6 to 10 seconds, then relax. Repeat five times.

The Pelvic Tilt can be done in a standing position or while seated at a desk or on an airplane as well, so it comes in handy all day long. It's also a terrific thing to do right before you hop (okay, crawl) into bed.

Flexion Routines

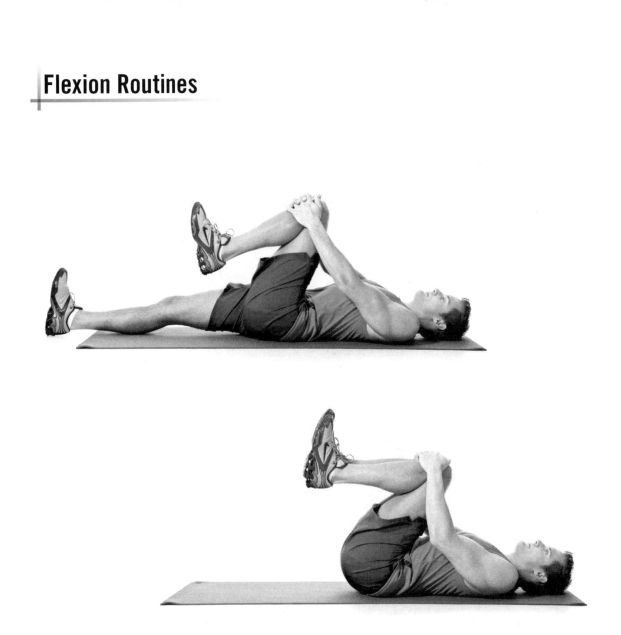

Knee-to-Chest

Start with the Pelvic Tilt and hold. Pull your left leg/knee toward your chest with your hands behind the knee area (or in front if that is more comfortable). Breathe gently and relax, keeping your head on the floor. Hold for 10 to 20 seconds, then repeat with your right leg.

Next, pull both knees to your chest. Relax and hold for 10 to 20 seconds. (If you are comfortable with these static positions, you can add a slight rocking motion.)

Repeat the sequence three or four times.

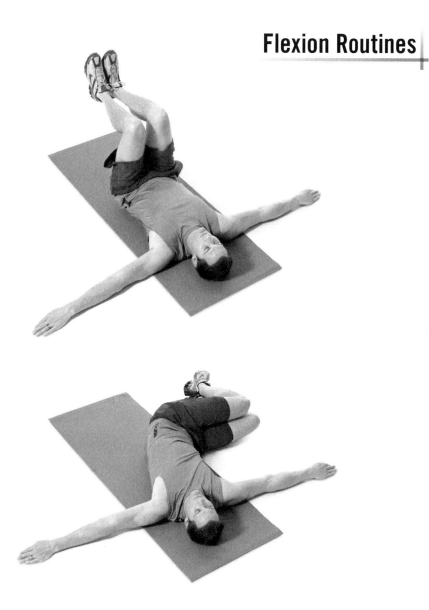

T-Roll

Lie on your back with your legs straight and arms stretched out to the sides so that you form a "T." Bring both of your knees up so that your hips and knees are flexed to 90 degrees. Keeping your palms, elbows, and shoulders on the floor and keeping your knees together, twist your torso and rotate your pelvis and knees so that your right knee is on the floor by your side. Hold for 5 to 7 seconds. Repeat on the opposite side. Repeat this sequence two times.

ACTIVE, NO MATTER WHAT

The National Center for Health Statistics says the incidence of neuromuscular conditions is on the rise, and that the increase may be linked in part to a combination of the increasingly sedentary lifestyle of Americans, the aging of our population, and the rise in obesity. The way things stand now, 80 percent of all people will experience lower back debilitation—knocked completely off their feet—at some point in their lives. The data is daunting, yes, but it can be an alarm that wakes us up to the fact that we need to focus more on our backs for better and longer-lasting health.

Dr. Mooney and other researchers discovered over the years that when back muscles are injured, they atrophy, and they develop strange fatty deposits, like a steak, that we really don't see in other injured muscle groups elsewhere in the body. Once your back's been injured, these muscles go on strike, getting caught in the trap of tightness, weakness, and malfunction. There's simply no alternative to doing lumbar exercises to get them back to normal.

Eighty percent of all people will experience lower back debilitation—knocked completely off their feet—at some point in their lives.

When it comes to back exercises, not all are created equal. If there is one muscle group that is the keystone to spinal support and resolving and/or preventing lower back issues, it is the lumbar extensor muscle group. Normal lumbar muscles (both the extensors and those transverse abdominal/oblique muscles responsible for rotation) not only are strong but also have a protective rapid response when needed for everything from simple twisting and bending to high-level sports activity.

I have learned a tremendous amount from Dr. Mooney regarding these unique muscles. When injured, or when associated with back pain, the lumbar extensors, especially the multifidus group, atrophy rapidly. This has been proven with CT imaging and MRI, and the more severe the back pain, the greater the degree of atrophy. Also, EMG (electromyogram) nerve testing has documented inhibition and malfunctioning of nerve firing patterns and function in these same muscles. The result is weaker muscles that fatigue more easily and don't respond as rapidly when they are needed.

This combination of weakness, low endurance, poor neuromuscular control, and sluggish response makes your back significantly more vulnerable. These findings are typical of someone who has had a back injury and is having persistent back pain and/or recurrent episodes.

These changes do not revert to normal on their own. The good news is that with specific targeted strengthening exercises, as outlined in Step 5, these abnormal findings can be completely *reversed* to normal. There are many other important muscles for optimal torso, core, and lower back function, but what I have learned from Dr. Mooney is that the lumbar extensors cannot be ignored if you want a healthy back.

To repeat: A back ailment is no excuse to avoid working out. People tend to think that painful symptoms are a bad thing, but they're not totally restrictive in the overriding majority of cases. What they are is a warning to "get your back up" about preserving your frame so it'll be there over the long haul.

Boomeritis: tendonitis, bursitis, arthritis, and . . . "fix-me-itis."

I've coined the term *Boomeritis,* which encompasses all of the aches and pains and musculoskeletal vulnerabilities that baby boomers have—tendonitis, bursitis, arthritis—and the "fix-me-itis" that goes along with them. Although baby boomers are the namesake of *Boomeritis,* they are not the only ones affected—no one is immune to these all-too-common musculoskeletal ailments. The best news is that, for the most part, getting "back" to health is in your hands. If the self-help approaches in this step don't get you past your back pain, there's a lot more in Step 6 that you can try before you offer yourself up for the instant gratification that you might think surgery provides. If you don't have one of those red flags listed earlier, the truth of the matter is that surgical intervention should be the absolute last resort.

Avoiding or mitigating back problems is in your hands, too, and I've got a bulletin for you: Your back muscles don't require a lot of extra work. All it takes are a few simple routines that you can incorporate into a regular exercise program. But before we take that step, it's time to find out what kind of shape your back is in right now.

Watch Your Back—Self-Test

If you're to be *active for life*, your back is going to play a big role. We can talk about aerobic fitness, about anaerobic fitness, but if lower back fitness doesn't match the level of either, you're not as fit as you can be. And that applies to everyone else who doesn't exercise at all and is happy to just get around without any problems. Because if you put some spine into your health *now*, you'll keep it in great shape to support you no matter what you do from now on.

As it should always be, before embarking on any exercise regimen, you must give pause. The simple test that follows will give you a gauge of just what shape your lower back is in. I know, I know—a lot of you would say, "Oh, it's all right," but I also know that means it stiffens or barks every now and then. This quiz will help you assess the health of your back so you can end pain now and prevent it in the future. Remember, no one is immune to lower back problems, and the lower back is the weak link in so many individuals' frames. You want to find your weak links before they find you! That way you can do something to prevent major breakdowns along the way. The good news is that even the beginner level program in Step 5 can make those pesky lower back reminders a thing of the past.

If you already have a lower back or other major joint limitation, by all means discuss the program in this book with your doctor before you do anything. Similarly, if you have a cardiac or cardiovascular condition, if you feel chest pain when you do physical activity, if you lose your balance because of dizziness, if you're taking prescription medication for blood pressure or your heart, or if you have any other major medical and/or orthopaedic issues or concerns, take the time to visit your doctor's office.

HEED YOUR WEAK LINK

You'll need about 30 minutes total for the self-test. You can breeze through the majority of the questions in about 5 minutes—just check the appropriate box (green/yellow/red) as you go along, and then you'll total each category at the end. Certain "red" responses are major warning signs, as they are especially predictive of ongoing or future back issues, and these have been starred. If you check any, be sure to discuss them with your doctor and proceed with caution in Step 5. A yellow response is a reminder that you could be doing better and/or there is something you need to improve upon or monitor. Green means smooth sailing. I've used this color-coded approach for many years with athletes, active individuals, and patients in my practice, and I know it gets to the heart of the matter very quickly. The 12 physical routines, however, will take up to half an hour. You should tackle them when you don't have any time pressure and are refreshed; and you'll need a friend for the last two of them, so you might want to schedule a separate time to complete that portion.

HISTORY

1. Do you have a family history of back problems?

a. No	green
b. Yes	yellow
c. Spinal surgery	red

2. Have you ever had lower back surgery?

a. No	green
b. It looms as a possibility	yellow
c. Yes	red*

3. If you are a woman, have you ever been pregnant?

a. Never	green
b. Yes, with no lower back issues	yellow
c. Yes—and with lower back issues that fully resolved after delivery	red*

4. Have you had to see a doctor or other health-care provider in the past 3 years for spine problems?

a. No	green
b. One or two visits, no problems most of the time	yellow
c. It's always on my calendar	red*

5. Do you have any stiffness in your lower back upon awakening (i.e., until showering or moving around for a while), after sitting still for more than 30 minutes, or for no apparent reason?

a. No	green
b. Only the day after a hard workout	yellow
c. It's a part of my life	red*

6. Have you ever had an episode of lower back or neck pain or spasm?

a. No	green
b. It kept me off my feet for less than 24 hours	yellow
c. I miss work because of recurrent episodes	red*

7. Do you find that you change your plans or activities because of your lower back?

a. No	green
b. Occasionally (no more than a few times a year)	yellow
c. Yes, my lower back is beginning to rule my life	red*

8. Do you have difficulty falling asleep at night or awaken during the night because of lower back discomfort?

a. No	green
b. Rarely or minor difficulty	yellow
c. It's a struggle as soon as my head hits the pillow	red

LIFESTYLE

1. Would you say you have a positive outlook on life?

a. Absolutely!	green
b. Depends on the day	yellow
c. How could anyone with all that's going on?	red

Body Mass Index Table

	Normal						Overweight					Obese									
BMI	19	20	21	22	23	24	25	26	27	28	29	30	31	32	33	34	35	36	37	38	39
Height (inches)																	**Body Weight (pounds)**				
58	91	96	100	105	110	115	119	124	129	134	138	143	148	153	158	162	167	172	177	181	186
59	94	99	104	109	114	119	124	128	133	138	143	148	153	158	163	168	173	178	183	188	193
60	97	102	107	112	118	123	128	133	138	143	148	153	158	163	168	174	179	184	189	194	199
61	100	106	111	116	122	127	132	137	143	148	153	158	164	169	174	180	185	190	195	201	206
62	104	109	115	120	126	131	136	142	147	153	158	164	169	175	180	186	191	196	202	207	213
63	107	113	118	124	130	135	141	146	152	158	163	169	175	180	186	191	197	203	208	214	220
64	110	116	122	128	134	140	145	151	157	163	169	174	180	186	192	197	204	209	215	221	227
65	114	120	126	132	138	144	150	156	162	168	174	180	186	192	198	204	210	216	222	228	234
66	118	124	130	136	142	148	155	161	167	173	179	186	192	198	204	210	216	223	229	235	241
67	121	127	134	140	146	153	159	166	172	178	185	191	198	204	211	217	223	230	236	242	249
68	125	131	138	144	151	158	164	171	177	184	190	197	203	210	216	223	230	236	243	249	256
69	128	135	142	149	155	162	169	176	182	189	196	203	209	216	223	230	236	243	250	257	263
70	132	139	146	153	160	167	174	181	188	195	202	209	216	222	229	236	243	250	257	264	271
71	136	143	150	157	165	172	179	186	193	200	208	215	222	229	236	243	250	257	265	272	279
72	140	147	154	162	169	177	184	191	199	206	213	221	228	235	242	250	258	265	272	279	287
73	144	151	159	166	174	182	189	197	204	212	219	227	235	242	250	257	265	272	280	288	295
74	148	155	163	171	179	186	194	202	210	218	225	233	241	249	256	264	272	280	287	295	303
75	152	160	168	176	184	192	200	208	216	224	232	240	248	256	264	272	279	287	295	303	311
76	156	164	172	180	189	197	205	213	221	230	238	246	254	263	271	279	287	295	304	312	320

Source: Adapted from *Clinical Guidelines on the Identification, Evaluation, and Treatment of Overweight and Obesity in Adults: The Evidence Report.*

Extreme Obesity

40	41	42	43	44	45	46	47	48	49	50	51	52	53	54
191	196	201	205	210	215	220	224	229	234	239	244	248	253	258
198	203	208	212	217	222	227	232	237	242	247	252	257	262	267
204	209	215	220	225	230	235	240	245	250	255	261	266	271	276
211	217	222	227	232	238	243	248	254	259	264	269	275	280	285
218	224	229	235	240	246	251	256	262	267	273	278	284	289	295
225	231	237	242	248	254	259	265	270	278	282	287	293	299	304
232	238	244	250	256	262	267	273	279	285	291	296	302	308	314
240	246	252	258	264	270	276	282	288	294	300	306	312	318	324
247	253	260	266	272	278	284	291	297	303	309	315	322	328	334
255	261	268	274	280	287	293	299	306	312	319	325	331	338	344
262	269	276	282	289	295	302	308	315	322	328	335	341	348	354
270	277	284	291	297	304	311	318	324	331	338	345	351	358	365
278	285	292	299	306	313	320	327	334	341	348	355	362	369	376
286	293	301	308	315	322	329	338	343	351	358	365	372	379	386
294	302	309	316	324	331	338	346	353	361	368	375	383	390	397
302	310	318	325	333	340	348	355	363	371	378	386	393	401	408
311	319	326	334	342	350	358	365	373	381	389	396	404	412	420
319	327	335	343	351	359	367	375	383	391	399	407	415	423	431
328	336	344	353	361	369	377	385	394	402	410	418	426	435	443

LIFESTYLE—*CONTINUED*

2. When you are under stress or stressed out, do you feel it in your lower back?

a. No	green
b. It's been known to happen	yellow
c. My lower back is hardwired to my brain	red

3. How stressful is your job and/or workplace?

a. Margaritaville—no or very little stress	green
b. Somewhat stressful but manageable	yellow
c. Major, out of control—I might as well be an air traffic controller at O'Hare or LaGuardia	red

4. Are you anxious and/or depressed?

a. No, pretty smooth sailing most of the time	green
b. Occasionally, but not too bad	yellow
c. Ongoing issue with me	red

5. Find your spot on the BMI chart on pages 50–51—are you significantly overweight?

a. Good weight (BMI below 25)	green
b. Mild overweight (BMI 25 to 29.9)	yellow
c. Overweight and/or obese (BMI 30 or over)	red*

6. Have you ever smoked?

a. No	green
b. Not in the past 10 years	yellow
c. I'm planning to quit	red*

7. What's your daily consumption of fruits and vegetables?

a. Seven to nine servings and a rainbow of colors	green
b. Maybe a green salad with dinner	yellow
c. Does ketchup qualify as a vegetable?	red

8. How often do you eat oily, cold-water fish, such as salmon or sardines?

a. Once or twice a week	green
b. A couple of times a month	yellow
c. Do Cheddar Goldfish cracker snacks count?	red

9. Do you take a daily vitamin and also sufficient antioxidants?

a. Never miss a day	green
b. I could be more consistent	yellow
c. Who has the time?	red

10. Do you consistently get adequate amounts of calcium and vitamin D (especially D$_3$/cholecalciferol)?

a. Yes, through my diet, supplements, and adequate sunshine exposure	green
b. Hit and miss	yellow
c. I thought "Got Milk" was for kids, and I rarely get outdoors, especially in the winter months	red

11. Do you routinely need to take over-the-counter medications, such as ibuprofen or naproxen, or prescription drugs for back discomfort?

a. No	green
b. Once or twice a month	yellow
c. I make sure to never run out	red*

12. Do you have to take prescription narcotic drugs for back pain?

a. No	green
b. On rare occasions (i.e., once or twice a year)	yellow
c. Pretty regularly, but have gone months without	red

13. How much water do you take in a day?

a. Eight full glasses	green
b. Four to six glasses, usually	yellow
c. I'm more of a camel—I go extended periods without a sip	red

14. For how many hours at a stretch do you sit at a desk?

a. Less than 2	green
b. 2 to 4	yellow
c. More than 4	red

15. How often do you work out?

a. Three times a week, an hour a day	green
b. Maybe once or twice a week	yellow
c. I've been meaning to join a gym	red

16. What does your workout consist of?

a. Balanced routines including aerobic, strengthening, stretching, and core work	green
b. A little of this and a little of that	yellow
c. Just one thing (running, yoga, swimming, weights)	red

17. How much sleep do you get each night?

a. 6 to 8 hours	green
b. 1 hour over or under that span	yellow
c. A lot more (or a lot less)	red

18. Is your sleep restful?

a. I can't wait to face each day	green
b. I often wake up tired, and some afternoons really drag	yellow
c. I check the clock during the night a lot more than I'd like	red

19. How do you usually pick up things off the floor (anything from a feather to a heavier weight—but especially the lighter things)?

a. I always "square up" to the object and, keeping my back pretty straight and upright, bend my knees	green
b. I bend my knees a little and bend over forward using my back	yellow
c. My knees are pretty straight, and I bend my back like a crane	red

GET PHYSICAL

Take your time to go through the checks below. If something—anything—is too demanding, or if it causes significant discomfort, *stop*. Circle any score that applies, and take a 2- to 3-minute breather. In any case, take a breather after every component, and don't go on until you're completely comfortable to do so. If you are unable to do a particular test because of discomfort, give yourself a "d" response for that question. It will still be important in the final tally.

1. Leg Length

Lie facedown (you'll need a friend for this) on a bed with only your feet and ankles hanging off (toes pointing down, legs straight, and feet together), and have your friend look down at your heels. (This is sometimes easier to see with shoes or sneakers on.) How are your heels aligned?

a. They are flush together and form a continuous surface	green
b. They are less than 1 centimeter off	yellow
c. They are more than 1 centimeter off	red

2. Lower Leg Strength

With knees splayed out like you are on a very large horse or small hippo, go into a partial squat (knees bent not quite to 90 degrees). Look straight ahead and hold this position up to 90 seconds. (If you are unable to do the "horse," try doing the "wall seat," which is an easier version.) How was your "ride"?

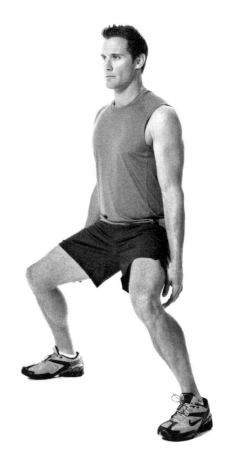

a. Can hold for 90 seconds then rise easily; actually found it a little relaxing	green
b. Struggled some, I could get down fine, but getting up was hard, or I could hold for 30 seconds, but my legs, they were a-shakin'!	yellow
c. You won't see me at the Kentucky Derby, 'cause I can't ride that horse hardly at all	red

3. Hip Tightness

Lie on a stable tabletop with your knees and lower legs hanging over the end. Bring both of your knees up until they are clutched to your chest in a "cannonball" position. Now, while one leg remains snug in that position, slowly lower the other. You should be able to place this other knee back fully flat on the table with your leg once again dangling over the side without your other hip coming down or your pelvis rocking forward. If it "hangs up," the front of your hip is too tight. Repeat with your other leg. How does it go?

a. Legs go back down fully, easily	green
b. Legs go back down fully, but feels tight in front	yellow
c. Leg or legs do not go down fully	red

4. Core Strength and Flexibility (Caution: If you are currently having back pain or have chronic recurrent episodes, skip this exercise.)

Lie down on that same table or on the floor, then tilt your pelvis so that you flatten your back as much as you can while drawing in and tightening your abdominal area. Now, with your legs perfectly straight, slowly raise your heels off the ground, then keep going as far as you can without discomfort, ideally until you reach 90 degrees to the hip (feet straight up). How far can you slowly, and in a controlled manner, bring your legs down toward the floor (while keeping them perfectly straight) before you have to arch your back (i.e., you're no longer able to keep your lower back flattened against the ground)?

a. Easy up and all the way back down in good form	green
b. Got 75 to 80 percent down in good form, then back area tilts, or it's difficult but I'm able to do it without discomfort or back arching	yellow
c. Can't perform test because of discomfort, or lower back tilts early on the way down	red

5. Core Strength and Endurance (Quadruped, see page 124)

While kneeling on the floor, place your hands flat on the ground as if you were to do a modified pushup. Next, assume the "plank" position, with your body straight and your full weight supported on both forearms and toes for 60 seconds. Next, lift your right arm off the ground for 15 seconds, supporting your full weight on your left arm and both feet. Repeat with your left arm, maintaining proper form.

Raise your right leg for 15 seconds, then return it to the ground and repeat with your left leg. Next, try to elevate your right arm and left leg simultaneously and hold for 15 seconds, then return them to the ground and repeat with your left arm and right leg. Return to the starting plank position and hold for an additional 30 seconds. How did it go?

a. Able to do all positions for the required time	green
b. Able to do all positions for half of the required time	yellow
c. Unable to hold all or any positions other than briefly	red*

6. Side Plank

Start on the floor lying on your left side, propping yourself up on your left forearm with your left elbow in line with your left shoulder, and your left outer thigh and leg on the ground with your feet lying stacked on one another. Your right arm should rest relaxed along your right side with your palm on your right hip. Press your hips toward the ceiling and lift your body off the floor to form a straight line, while balancing on your forearm and the side of your foot. Hold this position while contracting your abdominals to stabilize your torso. Breathe comfortably and don't hold your breath. Try to simultaneously tighten your abs and gluteal (butt) muscles, but keep your shoulders relaxed. Time yourself as you hold this position as long as you can comfortably without sagging or squirming. Now try this on the opposite side. How long could you hold?

a. 3 minutes	green
b. Less than 2 minutes	yellow
c. Less than 30 seconds or can't do	red

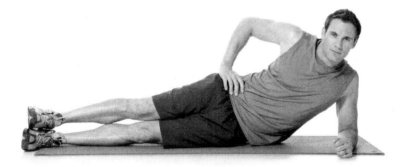

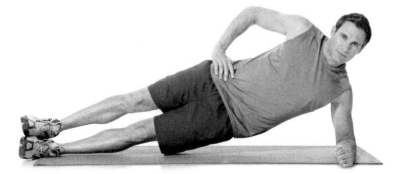

7. Hamstring (Back of Thigh) Tightness

Sit on the floor with your feet flat against a wall, with your feet pointing upward and your ankles at 90-degree angles. Sit tall (as if a string were pulling the top of your head toward the ceiling) and reach forward, with your index fingers touching side by side. While staying tall and keeping your chest high, slowly lean forward, keeping your knees straight, and try to touch the wall at the level of your eyes; i.e., don't reach down toward your toes but stay tall with good sitting posture. How did you do?

a. Can place both palms on the wall	green
b. Can reach the wall only with fingertips	yellow
c. Can't reach the wall	red*

8. Back Rotation

Lie on your back on the floor with your arms fully extended out to your sides, palms down. Pressing your hands against the floor, bring your left knee up and rotate it over your right leg. Without your left elbow, wrist, and shoulder coming off the floor, can you make your left knee touch the floor? Repeat with your right knee. How did you do?

a. Could touch the floor with both knees	green
b. Could get within 2 inches of the floor with both knees	yellow
c. Could not get within 2 inches of the floor with one or both knees	red

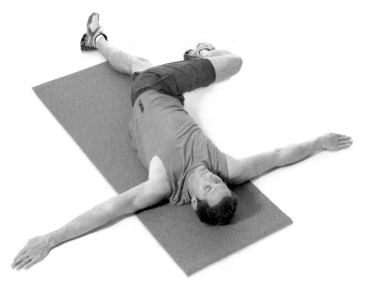

9. Abdominal Strength Crunches

Lie on the floor with your knees bent, your feet flat on the floor, and your arms crossed on your chest. Pull in and tighten your stomach, push your back flat, and rise high enough for your upper back to slowly come off the floor. Don't pull with your neck or head, and keep your lower back on the floor. How many crunches can you do slowly and with good form (i.e., 2 to 3 seconds up, brief pause, and 2 to 3 seconds down)?

a. More than 40	green
b. 25 to 40	yellow
c. Less than 25	red

10. Superman

Start by lying on the floor facedown with your arms straight out in line with your legs (picture Superman flying in the air). Raise both arms and legs off the floor; keep your knees straight so that your legs are being lifted by your buttocks and lower back. If it does not bother your neck, your head should also come off the floor. Hold for 10 seconds; if successful, build up to 30 seconds. Repeat with only your right arm and left leg raised. How did you do?

a. No problems at 30 seconds with either combination	green
b. 10 seconds was okay; couldn't make 30	yellow
c. Couldn't make 10 seconds	red*

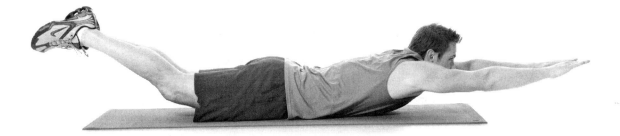

11. Posture

This is about how you carry your body—or your body carries you—and how you present yourself to the world. Wearing some tights or your underwear, have your partner snap a picture of you from the side while you stand as you naturally would (it's best if the photo is taken when you least expect it). Then place a ruler over the photo and draw a line from the back of your ear to your heel. Ideally, the line should bisect your shoulder, pass through your hip, and graze the back of your leg at the knee. How does your image look?

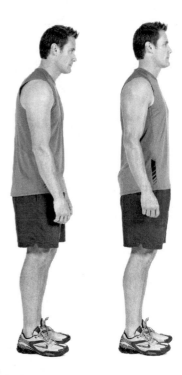

a. Straight as a soldier	green
b. A little stooped	yellow
c. Gee, I didn't think I resembled the Hunchback of Notre Dame	red

Now, have a photo taken—again, when least expected—while sitting naturally on a straight-backed, armless chair. This photo could best be described as:

a. The epitome of good posture	green
b. A bit bent over, but that usually is only when I am tired	yellow
c. Call me Slouch	red

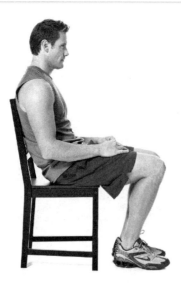
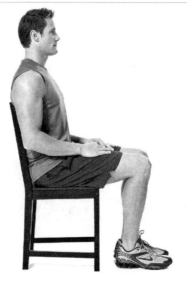

The above self-evaluation is not so much about a particular "score," it's about focusing on the critical issues and aspects of your life so you can lead a more active one. It's less about whether you have passed or failed and more about raising your awareness about the many things that contribute to having a healthy spine. The more "reds" you have, the more risk you have related to your lower back. What's most important, however, is that any weak links you have are modifiable, albeit some more easily than others. As you read this book, you will understand why these particular items were included in the self-test. You can strengthen or even resolve a weak link, make yourself far less vulnerable down the road, and toss "I threw my back out" into the dustbin.

Although everyone's case is unique, there are some general guidelines for which level of the FrameWork Lower Back Program is most appropriate for you.

Beginner/Recovery

As was mentioned earlier, everyone should start at this level because starting slowly is always indicated whenever new exercises are introduced into a fitness program. If you checked off any red boxes that have an aster-isk, consider yourself in serious rehab and plan to stay at this level for as long as it takes to resolve those issues or to manage them with your physician. If you checked a couple of lesser reds and/or mostly yellows, you should be able to move up within a month.

Intermediate

If you didn't check any reds but several responses were in the yellow category, you're likely mobile enough to get really serious about shoring up your lower back frame. Be faithful to the exercises at this level, and don't be surprised if you're a new person in 3 to 6 months.

Advanced

This is the level that most should aspire to. If your score included only a couple of yellows, you're probably the "fluid" sort who exercises or engages in recreational sport on a regular basis. At this level, you're in good shape for a future that is most rewarding.

High Performance

All green responses means you aced the test. You're an athlete or a fitness buff (or fanatic, as the case might be), and you'll attain new performance heights with this program as part of your overall regimen.

STEP UP

How'd you do? Are you a likely candidate for a "back attack"? Even if you're in the Rehab range and likely have some chronic lower back issues that significantly restrict your movement, you can do something *now* to end back problems, or at least live with them a whole lot better. It may take you a little longer to add some spine to your health, but, trust me, you'll get there, and you'll be amazed at how little you have to do to feel markedly better. You'll start off like everybody else with the next step and stay there until your body tells you to move on. When you start seeing a little more mobility after only a couple of days of the 10-minute warmup routine in Step 4, you'll realize that it's going to take you a lot less time than you thought to take the next step.

BACK TO THE START

Now you know all about your back and what can go wrong with it, and you've brought your weak links into sharper focus. But before you do any of the lower back routines in the next step that will put some spine into your health, you have to be sure you don't ignite a back episode or make your back a lot worse. Although exercise is a fantastic prescription for health, you have to do it right or it could be as harmful as, or even more harmful than, doing nothing at all.

A major study showed that one-third of exercisers had to drop out of a very conservative, medically supervised fitness program because of a musculoskeletal ailment—a frame injury—that cropped up. Your regimen might be great on the merits, but it might not be great for *your* frame. Most of the patients I see are committed to regular exercise, but approximately 80 percent need to revise their program because it overworks or underworks one or more vulnerable or potentially vulnerable areas. From the most tentative participant to the most seasoned workout fanatic, I find that something about their program just isn't right. The satisfaction I get from their efforts is tempered by the worry that they'll injure themselves and discontinue one of the very best things they can do for their health.

Even if you breezed through the physical tests in the previous step, you must not embark on a demanding lower back program if you don't have all of your ducks lined up properly. This means you have to be fit in general, and that requires a lot more than a weekly golf or tennis date, or occasional visits to a gym. You have to incorporate the four aspects of the FrameWork approach that complement targeted exercise and are just as vital for it: aerobic fitness, active rest and recovery, nutrition, and mind-body connection. If you internalize and use the information that follows, you won't miss a step when your lower back workout starts in earnest. In a sense, you have to take a step back before you take a major leap forward.

HEAVY BREATHING

Any program to improve overall health must include, at a minimum, aerobic exercise three times per week for 30 minutes, and your lower back program is no exception. If your back isn't in tip-top shape, however, some aerobic activities are clearly better than others. (For the most part, your heart doesn't know the difference aerobically between running and swimming—but your frame does!)

Rowing machines and rowing ergometers, for example, put high stresses on the back because of the seated position, so I would not recommend them in balky-back circumstances. Running is a great aerobic activity when you don't have back problems, but when your back is out or problematic, it's not a good idea. Even if your back is trouble-free, running is an activity that can create imbalances; a lot of runners only like to run and will typically have great hearts, fantastic aerobic fitness, and very strong calves, but where they suffer is they usually have extremely tight hamstrings, a tight lower back, and relatively weak abdom-

inals, so they're set up for back problems. Their frames are out of balance in large part because of the disparities created by the repetitive act of running. And runners are not alone in this area—many sports and recreational activities can create imbalances in your frame that set you up for musculoskeletal problems, including lower back pain. If you're a runner and like to run, that's fine—as long as you cross-train to include some targeted stretching, strengthening, and core exercises to keep your lower back out of trouble.

Motion is lotion.

Walking is a back-friendly aerobic option, and swimming is fantastic—even when you have an acute back episode and are in a lot of pain, subacute back pain, or just the run-of-the-mill chronic backache. If you're not a swimmer, or it seems your lower back is just too sore for you to swim, water exercise can still be very therapeutic. Try water walking, water jogging, or even water aerobics. If those activities aren't your cup of tea, take a bicycle to work or to the store, or just take it for a ride around your neighborhood. In the end, it doesn't matter what you choose to do as long as you get your heart pumping and your blood flowing, without causing harm to any part of your frame.

Poor aerobic fitness is a predictor of lower back episodes. There was a landmark study done involving firefighters out on disability claims, and it showed that the ones who had the worst aerobic fitness were more likely to miss work from a lower back injury, and those who were most fit aerobically were much more protected. It's all about microcirculation—the body's tiny network of capillaries—and the aerobic flush that gets the blood flowing. Your disks don't have a tremendous blood supply to begin with, and they're nourished by movement—motion is lotion, so to speak. Aerobic exercise helps your lower back in many other ways. By exercising, you keep your weight down, which lowers stresses on your spine. Also, through a release of endorphins and other systemic hormones, you lower stress, anxiety, and pain levels. So get your blood moving faster three times a week.

Smoke gets in your bones.

Antismoking messages are getting through to more and more people every day, but we still have to keep them coming. We'll "frame" the one here around bone health, how that nasty habit assaults the body's superstructure.

BACK STORY

When I was a resident in training, the hand surgeons were just starting to reattach severed fingers with microvascular surgery, known as replanting. That was the era when you actually could smoke in hospitals, and we would notice that if somebody was smoking a cigarette as he or she walked by the room of a patient who had had a replant, the reattached finger turned blue!

A while back, doctors discovered that smokers who underwent a spinal fusion weren't healing very well, to the point where many surgeons now say they won't do that procedure on someone unless he or she quits. They eventually linked poor bone healing with compromised bloodflow that results from vessel constriction caused by smoke inhalation. Smokers even have a higher incidence of lower back pain and lower back disk problems. We now know for sure something that had been suspected for a long time.

When I was in my orthopaedic surgical training at the University of Pennsylvania, Carl Brighton, MD, a brilliant researcher and the chief of my department, was doing research on

ARD

=====

tertion

Te Ching)

stretched

to its fullest capacity

may certainly snap.

A sword that is tempered

to its very sharpest

may easily be broken.

the microvascular small network of blood vessels. Incidentally, smokers have a higher incidence of shoulder rotator cuff injuries and spinal degenerative disk disease.

"ACTIVE" R & R

Fierce dedication to exercise is laudable, indeed, but proper recovery from exercise is a step that is often overlooked by many health-minded individuals. And if you're one of those who think that just alternating intense total-body workout activities—such as aerobic training one day, weight lifting the next—is adequate for recovery, you've got another thing coming, because your entire body needs to be shut down at times.

why some fractures don't heal—they're called delayed unions or non-unions—and there are a few bones in the body that are especially problematic. There were a lot more smokers hanging out in the waiting room in the "non-union" clinic where he worked a couple of days a week than at his regular orthopaedic practice, and smoking had something to do with the poorer bone healing he saw in the clinic.

As mentioned earlier, years later, many other doctors caught on to that, and it has to do with the fact that there are certain areas of the body where blood supply isn't great, and the body has to rely on its tiny network of capillaries. Smoking slows or prevents bone healing by constricting bloodflow. Even passive smoke exposure could instantly shut down

Overall stress accumulates in your body, and you aren't aware of that as you go on. Exercises might be directed at one area, but there is a cumulative toll on your system that can cause an overall crash or overuse injury. Overtraining syndrome and overuse injuries are preventable if you give your body the rest that it needs after bouts of heavier exercise.

Rest must occur both locally (for those certain muscles worked) and systemically (from an overall metabolic standpoint). Exercise is a powerful stimulus that creates spectacular changes in your body and frame, but those positive changes occur during the rest and recovery period. It is a critical time for making gains. Come back too soon and apply another stimulus before adequate recovery occurs, and you're asking for a breakdown. It's a lot like cell phones and PDAs—they have transformed how we live and how we communicate (or not), but if you don't routinely recharge the battery, they're useless. This applies to you, too. You must take time, and measures, to recharge.

This doesn't mean you should plop into a

BACKBOARD

Lesson: "Active" R & R Warning Signs

SYSTEMIC

Irritability, depression

Loss of drive

Loss of appetite

Elevated morning pulse rate

Sleep disturbance

Unexplained fatigue

Drop in performance

Workout plateau or halt in gains

LOCAL

Persistent muscle soreness

Overuse injury (tennis elbow, rotator cuff, jumper's knee, stress fractures)

recliner and put your feet up. There are better ways to recover from exercise:

- Casual walking
- Stretching
- Yoga
- Meditation

In other words, you can still "do" something (that's why we call it "active" R & R) to gain the benefit of doing nothing, like plopping into that recliner, which, by the way, is an acceptable option sometimes.

Your nutritional choices (covered in depth in the next section) are also very important in terms of recovery, especially after a hard workout or a few hours of your favorite sport. Muscle recovery is aided by taking in food, drink, or a supplement that contains the right mix of proteins and carbs within 30 minutes of stopping the activity. Interestingly, low-fat chocolate milk has been shown to be the perfect blend to aid and optimize recovery. (You should also refuel your muscles later that day with a quality high-carb meal.)

The importance of hydration cannot be overstated. It plays a critical role in helping your frame bounce back from the natural wear and tear that exercise causes. Water intake all day long and before, during, and after exercise is a must, because it oils your body's repair mechanisms.

Last, but not least, proper sleep is critical for recovery. Studies show that those who sleep less than 6 hours or more than 9 have impaired mental function, are more susceptible to disease, and have higher mortality rates. Prolonged periods of sleep unrest require the attention of a physician. If you are not among the 40 million of those who have a chronic sleep disorder, but you have an occasional bout with sleep disturbance (including snoring, a sign of low-quality sleep), there are some supplements you can take on a temporary basis to get you through (see Backboard on page 70 for specifics), and light exercise an hour before bedtime is a natural soporific (aka sleep remedy).

**Leave your work at work!
Invest in a good, comfortable mattress.
Read just before bedtime—no TV.**

The lowdown on your lower back fitness program is the same as that of any other exercise program: Gains in strength, flexibility, durability, and balance happen in your downtime. So take a day (or even two) off, but stay active in other ways and make proper sleep a priority.

YOU ARE WHAT YOU JUST ATE

When it comes to frame health, there are two issues associated with food: weight management and nutritional value. As 65 percent of us are either obese or overweight, we'll tackle avoirdupois first.

For every pound you carry, your hip and knee think it's 5 (or more, depending on your type of activity) because of load stresses, so if you're 10 pounds overweight, it feels like 50 to your frame! Excess pounds amplified in your frame cause and accelerate damage; they strain connective tissue, grind joints, and play a role in arthritis and other inflammation throughout your body.

The good news about poundage is that it works both ways—if you lose 5 pounds, your frame thinks you lost 25. But losing weight is one thing; keeping it off is quite another, and that's the primary drawback of otherwise excellent diet programs. They simply do not emphasize enough the critical ingredient in any diet: exercise. It's not that the value of exercise isn't known, it's that it's the elephant in the room that nobody wants to talk about. We're all too busy—and sedentary as a rule in our leisure time, albeit with the best intentions to work out regularly "someday."

Whether or not you're overweight, I'm here

to tell you that "someday" must be *today* because of the way metabolism works. It was programmed way back in our evolution as a survival mechanism. If you diet and significantly cut back on calories consumed, your body senses starvation and plays a nasty trick on you: It starts to cannibalize muscle first, not fat. Muscles use a lot of calories, so a loss of muscle mass lowers your metabolic rate, resulting in fewer calories burned. That makes you hungry, and you're more vulnerable to gaining weight with body fat because calories are first converted to fat. You can short-circuit this vicious cycle, however, with muscle building and toning.

Complicating matters is the fact that you will gradually lose muscle and weaken your frame as you age. That's why we're prone to weight gain as we get older. So, everyone, no matter how heavy or how old, has to exercise. Working out maintains and builds muscle, and that's what helps keep any excess weight

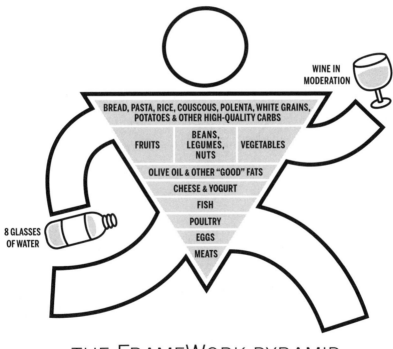

THE FRAMEWORK PYRAMID

The FrameWork pyramid stresses the importance of exercise, nutrition, and the role of the mind in creating and maintaining health. It's what you eat, what eats you, and what you do (or don't do) regularly that makes the difference.

off the frame. With every bit of muscle you add, you raise your metabolic rate and burn more calories, even if you're just sitting around doing nothing. So, pump some iron!

As for a weight-loss diet, the primary factor is calorie control. Science tells us that a pound is equivalent to 3,500 calories, so if your goal is to lose a pound a week, calorie intake must be reduced by 500 calories each day (or you must *burn* an extra 500 calories a day). Most rapid-weight-loss programs deprive the body of important nutrients, and the weight that is lost rapidly is usually water and muscle. Not good! The goal is to lose fat and get more lean.

Now that you know this, it's a matter of calculating exactly what you consume over a week, which is not all that tough to do when you consider the almost-universal labeling nowadays. So keep a running tab of *everything* you put into your mouth over 7 days, without changing your usual eating routine. Whatever that number turns out to be, divide it by 7, subtract 500, and that's your daily allotment that guarantees you will lose weight. (I'll let you in on a little secret: Your 500-calorie reduction doesn't have to come solely from giving up some food. That's a good thing, because if you're like me, you cherish every bite you take and might have a really tough time doing with-

BACKBOARD

Lesson: Temporary Sleep Supplements

5-hydroxytryptophan, or 5-HTP (50 milligrams)

Melatonin (3 milligrams)

Calcium (300 milligrams)

Magnesium (500 milligrams)

Valerian (400 milligrams)

out some favorites. Exercise of any kind burns calories in varying degrees; 20 minutes of walking makes about 50 calories disappear, 20 minutes of vigorous gardening lops off 75, and the same time spent doing strenuous aerobics burns 150 or more.)

There really isn't any magic involved in slimming down. It has nothing to do with a narrow focus on low carbs, all protein, good fats, or the new fad that either starves you or bores you to tears. It's about watching what you eat, and taking advantage of the excellent nutrition in all food groups. I recommend the Mediterranean Diet because it has everything you need and never bores the taste buds or the stomach. There are others that are balanced with good carbs, friendly fats, and anti-inflammatory foods, so eat whatever you

BACKBOARD

like—up to your limit and in proportion with the FrameWork Pyramid.

YOUR FRAMEWORK SMORGASBORD

This brings us to the other food issue: nutritional value. If you are what you just ate, you will be what you eat from now on. Again, you can choose what you eat, but you must choose wisely. You must include in your diet every major food group and every color of the rainbow. I'll leave the specifics about a menu up to you, but I have some general guidelines that will help you to eat in a healthy way.

A good rule of thumb is to allocate 20 percent of your diet to protein, 15 percent to polyunsaturated fats, 10 percent to monounsaturated fats, and 55 percent to good carbs. When you make your choices from these categories, give the nod every time to the ones highest in fiber content. (Very few among us, indeed, get the 25 grams per day that is optimal for weight and blood glucose control.)

Muscles require amino acids, those protein building blocks. Protein needs increase with age because of the associated muscle loss, and protein is always necessary to replenish muscle fiber. And yet protein is not as well absorbed into your system as you get older. The fact is, young or old, most of us do not take in enough protein. Why? Because we've all been cutting way back on red meat and eggs to reduce the risk of cardiovascular disease, and we haven't substituted enough of the better protein choices to make up the difference. Look for lean protein: chicken and turkey without the skin and salt (and hold the mayo, too), wild salmon, trout, herring, anchovies, and sardines, or soy if you're a vegetarian. Mix in some nuts, beans, and lentils to make up any protein shortfall.

We've all been warned about the dangers associated with butter, cheese, cream, and whole milk, but make sure some of your menu choices include good fats. The medical literature is peppered with studies that confirm the efficacy of the omega-3 fatty acids in olive oil, oily fish, nuts, and seeds—staples of the Mediterranean Diet. They are a boon to cardiovascular health, but they come with an advisory: Fats are extremely high in calories—200 in only $\frac{1}{4}$ cup of some nuts, for example—so measure quantities very carefully. The upside is that a small amount goes a long way to curbing your appetite. (Try a couple of tablespoons of hummus with half of a whole wheat pita, or a sliced banana with some flaxseed sprinkled on it, as an appetizer or snack and see for yourself.)

Good diets eliminate the carbs that aren't good for us—fried potatoes, white bread, white rice, sugar—but the best diet is loaded with carbs that fuel your frame while they fill your stomach—whole grains, leafy vegetables, fruit, and seeds. You don't have to totally give up bread and pasta, just make them a special treat or make sure they have the right ingredients. And, yes, you can indulge in the nutrition-rich potato—as long as it's boiled, steamed, or baked. Remember: The main fuel

BACKBOARD

Lesson: Good Carbs

Whole grain bread, cereal, and pasta

Brown rice, couscous, chickpeas, lentils

Oat bran

Leafy vegetables

Seeds (pumpkin, sesame, sunflower, flax)

Fruit (especially pineapple, grapefruit, cherries, unsweetened strawberries, peaches, and cantaloupe)

of choice for Olympic athletes is carbs. It really makes no sense to me when individuals who want to get fit, and look better, cut out carbs completely. For them I have two words: Michael Phelps. When training, he consumes over 12,000 carb-loaded calories a day!

Next on the FrameWork menu are foods that minimize inflammation and oxidation. It's no coincidence that the protein, friendly fats, and good carbs discussed above not only provide the right, balanced nutrition but also decrease inflammatory and cell-destructive reactions in your body. You might have noticed that junk food, fried food, saturated and partially hydrogenated fats, bakery goods, and sweets were nowhere to be found in the diet recommendations here. These food selections should be

BACKBOARD

Lesson: Friendly Fats

POLYUNSATURATED

Safflower, sunflower, corn, soybean oils

Walnuts

Oily fish

MONOUNSATURATED

Extra-virgin olive oil and canola oil

Avocados

Peanuts, hazelnuts, almonds, cashews

avoided like the plague because of the systemic havoc they wreak in your body. They promote inflammation, which can be destructive to both your heart and your frame. It is no wonder that the Mediterranean Diet is recommended for individuals with arthritis, since it is packed with anti-inflammatory nutrients.

Accent your menu with a wide variety of spices that don't add calories to your plate and that make your food tastier as they deliver antioxidation and anti-inflammation support.

Last, but not least, is a word about hydration. Water makes digestion possible; it is a solvent for nutrients and transports them everywhere. It assists muscle contraction and serves as a shock absorber all over your body,

especially in those disks between vertebrae. Water regulates your body temperature and eliminates waste products. And, for all you weight battlers out there, it fills you up and neutralizes food cravings.

Your blood is 90 percent water, your brain is 85 percent water, your muscles are 72 percent water, and your skin is 71 percent water. A water deficiency shows up as reduced mental acuity, fatigue, wrinkled skin, or the muscle cramps that both professional athletes and regular folks get sometimes when engaging in sports. If you feel plumb tuckered out, have a headache or eyestrain, or have sore muscles in your neck and back, it might have nothing at all to do with overwork and stress—it just might be a serious lack of aqua.

Bottom line? You need to drink 2 quarts of water every day. As it is with fiber, however, few among us consume that much. So be like one of those people we see all around who have a water bottle in their hand, cup holder, or carryall, or on their desk. (Drinks that contain caffeine don't count—caffeine is a diuretic that drains body fluid. If you've had your fill of water, try grape, cherry, acai, goji, or pomegranate juice; teas, especially green tea, that don't contain caffeine; or smoothies made in a blender using fruit, ice, and low-fat yogurt.)

BACKBOARD

Lesson: Supplements for a Healthy Spine ("Vita-musts")

Multivitamin

Antioxidants (vitamins A, C, and E)

Calcium and vitamin D_3

Omega-3s

Cosamin ASU* (if arthritis is a factor)

*contains glucosamine, chondroitin sulfate, avocado, soy, and green tea extract

SUPPLEMENTAL NUTRITIONAL ADVICE

Even if you eat all the best things all the time, your gastrointestinal system is inefficient—it can't extract all of the good nutrients from the food you ingest. That, coupled with taste preferences that may inadvertently be causing you to miss out on something your frame needs, is why every diet must include some basic over-the-counter supplements. (Beware, you bargain shoppers out there: Supplements, unlike pharmaceutical-grade drugs, do not have to meet label claims. Many companies use foreign suppliers whose ingredients have less-than-advertised potency, and some use additional substances not on the label that could be quite harmful to you, especially if you are taking any prescription medication. The brand matters—buy only from reputable manufacturers that conform to strict codes regarding prod-

BACK STORY

Calcium and vitamin D are well-known for their important role in building bones and preventing osteoporosis. Recent research has also shown an important role in spine health and back pain prevention. Not only do they keep your spine's many bones strong, but vitamin D (specifically D_3, or cholecalciferol) has been shown to help with chronic back pain. Researchers found that significant percentages of chronic lower back pain sufferers are vitamin D deficient, and when adequate supplements (1,000 to 2,000 IU a day of vitamin D_3) were given, back symptoms vanished or at least improved in a majority of patients. Vitamin D is called the sunshine vitamin, because the body makes it when one has adequate exposure to the sun's ultraviolet rays. Many individuals are vitamin D deficient, especially because of the concerns about skin cancer and UV exposure, as well as a large segment of the population who remain indoors, especially in the winter months in cooler climates. I strongly recommend calcium and vitamin D_3 supplementation.

ASSIGNMENT: GET A RAINBOW OF NUTRITION

Red: Tomatoes, red peppers, pink grapefruit, watermelon

Purple: Blueberries, plums, beets, eggplant, red cabbage

Reddish orange: Carrots, mangoes, cantaloupe, winter squash, sweet potatoes

Yellow/orange: Peaches, papaya, nectarines, pineapple

Yellow/green: Spinach, corn, green peas, avocado, honeydew melon

Green: Broccoli, brussels sprouts, cabbage, kale, bok choy

White/green: Garlic, onions, leeks, celery, asparagus, pears, green grapes

uct quality and labeling. The best companies earn the United States Pharmacopeia [USP] seal of approval.)

In addition to including a broad-spectrum multivitamin (and calcium and vitamin D supplementation), a program that buttresses your diet and bolsters your frame covers three vital areas: bone/connective tissue support, antioxidant protection, and inflammation control. (Check the "Assignment" on page 77 for your supplement assignment.)

Digestive inefficiencies also explain in part those hunger pangs we get now and then. One trick of a diet that you can stick to is to split your daily protein allowance over two or three meals; protein takes longer to break down, so you feel full longer. Another trick is to allocate 20 to 40 percent of your daily calorie allowance to healthy snacks. Many people find having

multiple, smaller "meals" spread throughout the day keeps them satisfied and lessens the urge to binge at regular mealtimes. This approach also tends to keep blood sugar and insulin levels more stable throughout the day, which helps reduce systemic inflammation and lessens body fat production and storage. Get in the habit of having a plastic sandwich bag with some goodies handy so you don't end up with a soda or candy bar to satisfy a craving.

Yes, weight management and healthy nutrition come down to the choices you make every day about what you will put into your mouth—both quantity and quality. You'll either increase your fat, your blood sugar, and inflammatory reactions in your muscles and joints, or reduce them with the help of Mother Nature. Acquire better food habits and make better choices: extra-virgin olive oil and vine-

ASSIGNMENT: LIBERAL USE OF SALUTARY SPICES

Top 10 Antioxidant Condiments		Top 10 Anti-Inflammation Condiments	
Turmeric	Basil	Hot chile peppers	Basil
Cinnamon	Cumin	Ginger	Cloves
Oregano	Sage	Curry powder	Garlic
Cloves	Mustard seed	Black pepper	Parsley
Parsley	Marjoram	Rosemary	Onion

gar instead of Caesar salad dressing; teas and unsweetened juices instead of soda that blocks calcium absorption because of its phosphorus content; dark honey or stevia instead of sugar; mustard instead of mayonnaise; fresh food prepared fast instead of fast food. (And don't forget to grab a cup of water every chance you get.)

Eat well and have fun doing it. Enjoy that glass of red wine (or at least grape juice) as well. It's a great way to extend your frame's warranty.

CHILLING OUT

Sports medicine doctors know that psychological issues are important in dealing with orthopaedic problems and injuries. And yet history has shown that many, if not most, of us aren't very good at doing anything about them. There are times when I walk into an examination room, and before I even know what the patient's issue is, I have a feeling—a sixth sense—that I won't be able to help that person. I know that

BACK STORY

Resveratrol, a compound that is found in red grapes and red wine and has been touted for its potential benefits in improving longevity, also has anti-inflammatory properties. More recently, in an animal cell–culture study, it was shown to possibly hinder disk (remember those spongy shock absorbers in your spine) degeneration. Resveratrol was found to help both form and fortify proteoglycan, an important building block of the disk connective tissue. In terms of resveratrol supplements, I prefer Bioforte resveratrol by Biotivia (biotivia.com) because of its high potency and proven quality.

the right diagnosis and treatment won't be enough to get that person better because there are emotional or other psychosocial issues involved. That "baggage" hasn't been checked.

The mind affects how you feel and how you heal.

Orthopaedic specialists are aware of the importance of a patient's mind "frame." We've seen the same studies every other doctor has that unequivocally connect stress with immune dysfunction and disease, but we haven't connected all the dots on how to help patients who are stressed out. Mind and body are seen as two completely different and completely separate realms. We, as surgeons, all too often just deal with the physical; we don't get patients to the right person, or incorporate a team approach, or, perhaps most important of all, call on them to help themselves emotionally. The result is suboptimal healing and/or recovery and recurrent frame-related (or other) ailments.

That's beginning to change in a big way. Psychoneuroimmunology (PNI) is a medical discipline, still in its formative stages, that was established to clarify the complex hormonal and biochemical triggers that alter the immune response and other physiological systems. Either these triggers allow your mind and central nervous system to give you a boost, or they set off a downward spiral.

The connection between mind and body related to lower back ailments is remarkable. It's been documented beyond question that stress plays a major role in both acute and chronic pain. Researchers at Stanford University found that patients with poor coping skills were four times more likely to develop significant problems with their lower backs. In fact, psychological test scores were far more predictive of back problems than any structural abnormalities found on an MRI or other imaging! Other studies have shown that the best predictors of long-term work-related lower back disability have more to do with psychosocial factors like job performance and job satisfaction than any physical parameter.

Helen Flanders Dunbar, MD (1902–1959), an important early figure in US psychosomatic medicine and psychobiology, said, "It's not a question of whether an illness is physical or emotional, but how much of each." Simply stated, if we ignore the emotional side, we're not going to be as successful as we could be in getting people better.

In my experience, a significant number of doctors fail to appreciate this. So we see more

BACK STORY

When I was in med school, we knew pretty early in the training process who among our classmates was going to go into which specialty—some students had research-oriented personalities, others were inclined to a specific organ or other specialty, and others were best suited for general practice. There also seemed to be two extremes: orthopaedic surgeons, the "cowboys," the Mr. Fix-It, very hands-on mechanical types on one end, and those who wanted to go into psychiatry, the more analytical, ethereal, on the other. (We referred to their calling as "treatment of the id by the odd.") Back then we really thought we were at two *opposite* ends of the spectrum. It was only after being in practice for a period of time that I began to realize how close the two really are to each other, and how intertwined they are when it comes to keeping patients healthy and able to manage their medical conditions.

tests, more surgeries, more utilization of our already strained health system—not always to the advantage of the patient. This is especially true in spine care. Stress, anxiety, depression, and other emotional issues are often the elephant in the corner of the room that all are ignoring. Your doctor might see it, but he or she might not be comfortable dealing with it. You need to be honest with yourself and bring it up, even if it is only a potential factor. It may be one of the keys to getting you better and/or avoiding unnecessary treatment.

When it comes to psychological distress, clearly there is a wide range of severity. Anyone who is affected daily (work or relationship slippage) by any mind issue must seek professional help. If there are psychosocial issues in play in your case, talk to your doctor about possible interventions. I've heard, and I believe, that broken bodies are easier to heal than broken minds. Opening up and talking about these things is an important first step toward optimal healing and recovery. That's a big part of what the FrameWork back program is all about.

STARVE WHATEVER IT IS THAT'S EATING YOU

Doctors aren't the only ones not doing enough when it comes to mind frame—everyone bears some responsibility for how they feel and how that affects their health. You may not be able to do much about the circumstances that weigh upon you, but you sure can acknowledge they exist (don't bury your head in the sand about them), and you sure can do a lot to combat them.

■ RELAXATION BREATHING

Unconsciously, most of us take shallow breaths all day long, and that is the rule whenever we are in an excited or agitated state that actually produces or exacerbates stress. The following routine is so simple that you can do it anywhere, and it's something you should do a few times every day whether you're experiencing tension or not. *Do not force any movements, and remember to use slow, controlled movements.*

1. Straighten your spine and keep your eyes closed during all of the steps in this breathing routine. Rotate your neck slowly to the right and hold for 5 seconds; repeat to the left. Bend your chin forward toward your chest and hold for 5 seconds; bend your head back as far as it will go comfortably and hold for 5 seconds. Bend your head toward your right shoulder as far

as you can go and hold for 5 seconds; repeat to the left (again, within your comfort range).

2. Notice your regular breathing—feel it expanding your lungs, then emptying from your lungs.

3. Take deeper breaths and notice how the infusion of additional oxygen clears your head. Focus exclusively on this, driving everything else from your mind.

4. Take even deeper breaths slowly through your nose. Hold for 1 to 2 seconds. Release

BACK STORY

You may be familiar with the national retail chain Relax The Back, whose stated goal is to help people who are seeking relief from and prevention of back pain. I believe that this type of store offers tremendous educational and functional items for those with back pain, and I especially like their concept of relaxing the back. However, I have a slightly different sequence for those who want relief from back pain:

Relax the mind.
Work the back.
Then . . . relax the back.

the air through your mouth while relaxing your entire body. Repeat three times.

5. Breathe normally through your nose three times, focusing on the oxygen coming into your body and thinking about it expanding your chest, entering your bloodstream, and circulating from your forehead to your toes.

6. Continue taking slow, deep breaths through your nose, but now let your belly expand so that you're breathing with your diaphragm. When your lungs are full, hold the breath for 2 seconds. (Until you get this deeper breathing down, place your palms on your abdominal area and actually feel your abdomen expand.)

7. Release the breath slowly through your mouth and exhale until your lungs feel completely empty—contract your belly to force out every last air molecule. Wait 2 seconds.

8. Repeat the cycle three times, starting with step 4 above.

Once you get comfortable with this stress-busting routine (think "mental pushups"), you can do it anytime, anywhere. Also try it lying down on your back, or in bed at night with a pillow under your knees. Skip the neck exercises and just concentrate on the breathing. This type of mindfulness breathing can also be used to relax all of your muscles and even get added relief for your spinal area, a place where tension loves to hide.

ID YOUR STRESS BUTTONS

There are certain things (or people)—at home, at work, at school, even at play—that set your mind and body racing. You usually know what they are (if not, you need to start figuring it out), and you know when they kick in. What you might not know is that you can train yourself to switch off your brain as soon as one of these things occurs. You can make the conscious decision to distract your mind with a more pleasant or innocuous thought. Practice this—it works.

OPEN YOUR RELIEF VALVE

You also know what calms you down, what distracts you from whatever worries you have and gets you into the psychological state called "flow." Exercise, writing, and juggling work for me; whatever works for you—a leisurely stroll, model building, poker playing, listening to your playlist, frolicking with the kids—should be brought into play

BACK STORY

Right before every intense surgical session, I set aside a few moments to be alone with my breathing. It's something I learned with exposure over the years to martial arts, yoga, and meditation, which helps me "cool" my systems. A little time—less than 3 minutes, actually—focusing solely on the air entering and leaving my body, and I'm ready for anything that lies ahead. I'm relaxed, and my concentration is heightened.

whenever you need to let off steam. And, although you can't find it in any anatomy book, your "tickle bone" is an essential part of your frame—find it, and laugh your cares away every now and then.

TALK IT OFF

Keeping things bottled up can and will backfire with physical and emotional consequences. Talk to a friend, a significant other, or your doctor. Let things out; it helps. A recent study published in the *Archives of Internal Medicine* showed that participation in an e-mail discussion group was enough to help reduce pain and disability in individuals with chronic lower back

BACKBOARD

Lesson: De-stress

pain. So, please, talk . . . or should I say chat/text?

■ SOOTHE YOURSELF

There is a host of things that pacify just like Mom used to do (or still does, if you're fortunate to still have her with you). Listening to waves at the seashore or staring into a fire (and other repetitive nature sounds and images); taking a long, hot bath; massage; yoga; meditation; tai chi; progressive muscle relaxation (PMR—see "Backboard" assignment on page 83, and combine it with Relaxation Breathing); and hot tea or water with lemon all have remarkable salutary effects. Studies

have recently shown that certain "comfort foods" can actually dampen or reduce pain signals—but be careful not to overeat! Take every opportunity you can to nurture your mind frame.

■ THINK POSITIVE

It might not be in your nature to be optimistic, but its proven benefits are so huge that it pays to learn to suspend your disbelief or cynicism. Pick up a bestseller on this topic and adopt the approaches that are comfortable for you.

Guided imagery (used for centuries by yogis to control heart rate and body temperature) is a form of positive thinking. Studies have shown that an aquarium in a room can lower blood pressure and that conjuring a tranquil place or activity in your mind can have the same effect. Stay with the image, make it real, and don't be surprised if your tension eases.

"In Chinese medicine a symptom isn't something to eradicate, but a *message* about where we need more balance."—Dr. Frank Lipman

Along with the above approaches, here are a few others to keep stress in check:

- Eat right. (Food affects mood, as anyone who has witnessed a child after a sugar binge could tell you.)

- Hydrate, hydrate, hydrate. (We've discussed how the lack of water can strain your eyes, neck, and back—is it a surprise that these add to overall tension?)

- Stick to an exercise program and get proper sleep.

There are a lot of proven stress reducers to choose from here, but don't let that increase your anxiety. The only "must learn" strategy is the Relaxation Breathing because its calming effect not only cuts tension but prepares your frame for exercise—lower back or otherwise. As for the rest, choose wisely and incorporate everything that's appropriate to your circumstance and preference.

YOUR FRAME, FIT FOR ACTION

Does it make much sense to sign up for a marathon if you can't walk to the corner store without difficulty? Of course not. Likewise, it isn't prudent to vigorously train your lower back if your body and mind aren't in tune for that exercise, if you aren't fit in general. The four FrameWork components discussed in this chapter will go a long way toward getting you where you need to be; throw in the basics of

physical fitness, and you'll cross the finish line that is the starting point for the targeted routines in the next step.

Five or six 30- to 60-minute periods every week is all you need for your body to perform better, without pain or with a lot less of it. In addition to the aerobic exercise component discussed earlier, incorporate the two elements below as part of your FrameWork general fitness foundation. The first one you *must* do before you dash out the door in running attire, pick up a racket or golf club, hit the gym, or engage in any other physical activity.

- **WARM UP AND S-T-R-E-T-C-H**
  These are two different things. A warmup gets the blood flowing through

BACK STORY

Arnold Schwarzenegger has been my friend for many years, and I have learned so much from him about the power of a positive mind-set as it relates to both happiness and accomplishment. He is a master of putting positive thought to work.

Many years ago, during his days as a championship bodybuilder, Arnold talked about his mental concentration that directed more blood to specific muscle groups. His fellow athletes and most doctors thought he had gone around the bend, but subsequent biofeedback research on this example of guided imagery has proven him right.

your body and warms muscles and tendons so they'll behave more elastically. They'll be less likely to pull or tear, and this is especially true as you age or if you've had any injuries. Meanwhile, stretching allows the muscles to become more pliable and able to operate in a broader range of motion.

No professional athlete or serious fitness buff would ask his or her body to perform without a proper warmup. As a physician for professional athletes for many years, I have had the opportunity to arrive at the stadium hours before a sports event begins, and I can tell you firsthand that the athletes spend extensive amounts of time preparing their bodies for what's to come. They execute all of the movements required for their sport at reduced speed. We've

all seen the "weekend warriors" with a foot against a wall or on a bench, their hands stretching to their ankles or at their waists as their hips arc forward and back. They stand on one leg and grab a raised knee, they rotate at their hips with deliberate motion, they raise themselves up onto their toes. When they're finished, they're good to go.

Everyone else pretty much just grabs a racket, bag of clubs, Frisbee, or volleyball for an occasional foray into sports and feels lucky to be able to carve out enough time for the activity. "Fifteen minutes for a *whole routine* to loosen up?" these people ask. "That'd be nice, but . . . you know," they sigh. At most, they'll bounce on their feet or try to touch their toes once or twice. Stretching gets squeezed out, so to speak. To one's peril, I'll add.

This group is in the overwhelming majority who circumvent the most neglected area of exercise routines, thus explaining the preponderance of sprains and strains and pulls, the ligament tears, and the arthritis, that fill my calendar.

Muscle tightness is closely linked to specific injury patterns. This is especially true in individuals with chronic lower back issues who all too often have tight hamstrings, tight anterior (front) hip muscles, and a tight lower back. You need to warm up and stretch like the pros do (albeit with less intensity and duration) so your body can perform as it should and reap maximum benefit from whatever exercise you do. The routine described in Step 5 takes only a few minutes, but it makes such a huge difference that you might find yourself doing it at times other than exercise periods.

■ CORE STRENGTH AND FLEXIBILITY

A strong trunk is critical for balanced and optimal use of all musculature, and it lessens the chance for injury that comes when you strain to get power from just your arms or legs. Spend more time building up the muscles in the middle: back extensors (the "back" of the back),

abdominals (the "front" of the back), and oblique muscles (the "sides" of the back).

General physical fitness is protective for your lower back—the more fit you are, the less likely you are to have back issues. (For more in-depth information about the FrameWork philosophy and detailed comprehensive fitness and rehabilitation routines, please see Additional Resources on pages 167–68.

BACK YOURSELF UP

Want to know how to have a pain-free back? Take the next step—it's the "core" of your lower back program.

If you have any problems at first, don't give up. You probably had difficulty with some of the self-assessment exercises, too, but that's why you're here: to work out the kinks. As long as you don't have one of the red flags waving at you, you can proceed—very slowly.

Even if you can manage only one stretch or exercise, do it every day for a couple of weeks. If you can exercise only for a brief period of time, then do it several times per day. I'm betting you're still going to notice a significant improvement in range of motion and balance. Add more exercises and intensity at your own pace. Before you know it, you'll start catching yourself forgetting about a backache that always seemed to be with you. Durability—

BACK STORY

I'm one of those "beat-up" guys who have a full complement of creaking body parts after years of serious recreation. Tennis remains a passion, and if I didn't do the following "pre-match" routine religiously, I'd be on the sidelines a lot more.

- 30 jumping jacks
- Jogging in place for 2 minutes
- Rotational twists (10 on each side)
- Side bends (10 on each side)
- 20 toe touches
- 5 deep knee bends (I have to hold on to something because of a cranky knee.)
- Holding my racket, I go through tennis-specific movement patterns for 2 minutes to awaken muscle memory: forearm and calf stretches, windmills, low-intensity service motion, and practice swings.
- Gentle volleying from midcourt for a couple of minutes

I spend a scant 5 minutes off the court and about the same on it. In less than 10 minutes, I'm good to go.

---

and sustained improvement—will arrive soon after as the lower back exercises become easier over time.

The core is the epicenter of your frame.

There's no clock involved, and there's no shame in taking a side step if you need more time to master the stretches and initial exercises that follow. Remember, I said everyone can feel better. And that begins the moment you start with a purpose to work out.

If backache is a frequent companion of yours, it will become less familiar. If you're a tennis or basketball player, golfer, or volleyball aficionado, you will recreate better. Everyone will perform better, whether that's on an athletic field or at home. You can journey to the center of your core and build your back so it will stand up to a lot more movement and higher loads. That's how injury—and pain—are prevented.

Commit yourself to pushing yourself, and take the next step with confidence.

BACK IN SHAPE

By now you've taken significant steps in your path to spine health and you've learned a lot about your back. You've learned about its framework, how it breaks down, how it can be treated, and how it can be restored to health. Simple exercises were a critical part of your overall program. When you incorporate the more extensive exercises in this step, you'll find out just how powerful the medicine they deliver is.

Everything to this point is but a prelude to the transformation your body will undergo after you make focused back exercises a habit. We'll get to those soon, but before we do, let's make sure we're on the same page when it comes to being ready.

■ You discussed your intentions with your doctor, right? Let me emphasize once more that no treatment modality should be embarked upon without full disclosure to your primary physician and other appropriate health-care providers—especially those involved in the care of your lower back.

■ The FrameWork Lower Back Program doesn't exist in a vacuum—it is meant to be a part of a comprehensive, regular fitness regimen that maintains the entire frame, inside and out. That means a vigorous cardio workout three times per week for at least 30 minutes is included.

If you are among some of those whose limitations preclude vigorous or even moderate-intensity exercise, you get a pass here—for now. You should be able to do something, however, to get your body moving, even if it is low-intensity, shorter-duration bouts of exercise and/or activity throughout the day. As soon as you've mastered the first level in Step 5, however, you're expected to advance, both within the lower back program *and* to other routines outlined in *FrameWork* or another reputable fitness course.

■ As we covered earlier, a certain amount of discomfort, especially if you have an out-of-whack back, is to be expected when doing any physical activity. Trial and error comes into play again here. Listen to your body—if you think the pain you feel while trying an exercise is more intense than is manageable, skip it and move on to another, but remember the difference between hurt and harm, as discussed earlier. A little hurt is usually okay and sometimes must be worked through to get out of your physical rut. Your physician, chiropractor, or physical therapist can often help you distinguish between the two and reassure you, when needed, that no harm is being done.

■ Slow, controlled movement, not bouncing to and fro, is the cornerstone of safe, effective exercise routines. Never sacrifice form to get more reps or to use a heavier weight or resistance. And keep in mind there is significant benefit from both concentric (up) and eccentric (down) motions. Optimal balanced muscle growth and development require attention to both phases of the lift, up and down, whether it is a biceps curl or a lower back extension, as each builds the muscle differently. Both will increase endurance and build strong body parts, so don't cut yourself short when doing your lower back routine. Also, these exercises will be more effective if you use a mindfulness technique in which you stay focused and concentrate on the muscles being called upon during the movements. Lastly, incorporate relaxation-type breathing (see page 79).

READY, SET . . . HOLD ON A SEC

Odds are that by now you're champing at the bit to take your back out for a real spin. Truth is, that can't happen soon enough for me, but there are two considerations you should think about before you exercise in earnest.

■ **CARDIO-TYPE WARMUP**

As we covered in depth in Step 4, you have to get your blood moving before you exercise. Three to 5 minutes of jumping jacks, cycling, power walking, jogging, or marching in place is all it takes. The key is to break a light sweat—and this gets especially important as you progress to the higher levels of the lower back routines. Do it

BACKBOARD

Assignment: S-T-R-E-T-C-H

- Front of shoulders

- Lower back

- Hamstrings

- Calves

every time to avoid injury and get the most out of your lower back exercise.

■ S-T-R-E-T-C-H-I-N-G

This is a great idea anytime; it's indispensable prior to a workout. These targeted stretches are ideal for lower back maintenance and prevention. They can be done safely every day, or perhaps on cardio days (before and/or after the workout), especially for those who showed

significant tightness in the Step 3 self-test. They are an essential part of the pre–lower back exercise warmup after you have broken your sweat. For those of you who are strung particularly tight, try to stretch every day and follow the 3×30 stretching routine in which you hold each stretch for 30 seconds and do it three times. This has been shown to provide optimal stretching of tight muscle groups. Also, consider taking up yoga and get a copy of *Stretching* by Bob Anderson (Shelter Publications).

Remember that your lower back frame is connected to other parts of your body, and everything must work in concert. That's when back recovery is fastest and most effective—and when back health is maintained best. Spend a few minutes on the following routines and you'll reap maximum reward.

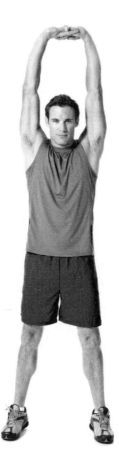

Pillar

Interlace your fingers in front of you, turn your palms outward, and then reach for the sky, palms up, until your hands are directly over your head with your elbows straight. Hold for 30 seconds.

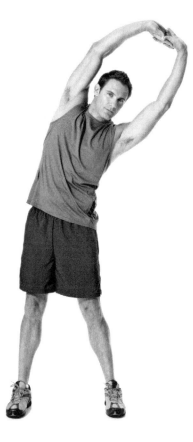

Pillar with Side Bend

With your hands and arms over your head as in the Pillar, lean
gently to your left and then to your right.

Stretching

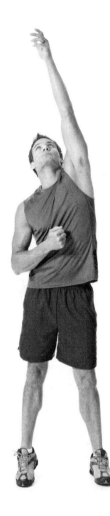

Climb the Rope

While looking up slightly, tighten your abdominal area by moving your belly button toward your spine. Reach up with your left hand, then reach even higher. Cross your right hand over the left as if you were climbing a rope (*really* reaching is important)—you should feel it in your shoulders, upper back, and abdominal obliques. Do 5 repetitions on each side.

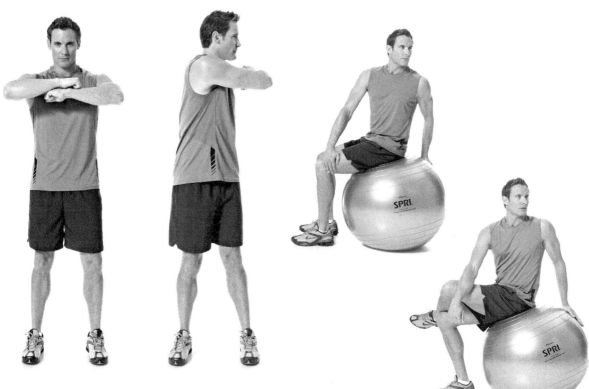

Standing Twist

Stand with your elbows up at shoulder height and abs tightened. Rotate right, then left, gently turning as far as possible to each side with each twist. When you reach your deepest twist, immediately reverse the movement and twist to the other side.

Or try this sitting on a gym ball: Sit tall and tighten your abs as above and place your right hand on the outer side of your left knee/thigh. Rotate at the spine to the left, gently pushing with your right hand to help turn your spine and shoulders. Look behind you and stretch your left arm as far as you can. Steady the ball with your left hand, if needed, to assist. Repeat with your left hand on your right knee. When on the ball, hold each twist for 5 to 7 seconds.

More advanced alternative: Sitting on the ball, do the twist with your legs crossed and your arm resting on the opposite knee area.

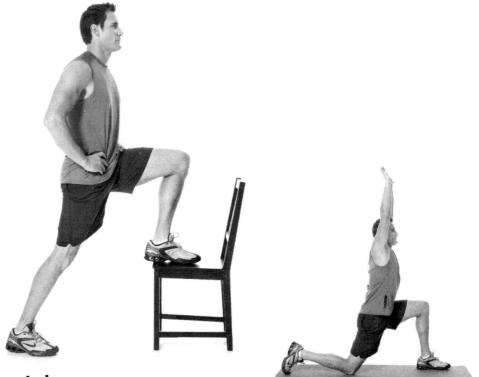

Psoas Stretch

Place your left foot flat on the top of a hard chair, stool, or step so that it is about 2 feet above the floor. Keep your right leg straight, with your foot pointing forward or slightly inward. Lean forward, keeping your back straight, until you feel a stretch in the front of your right hip. Hold for 20 seconds and then alternate sides. Rest for a minute or two and repeat.

Alternate Psoas Stretch:
Kneel on your right knee with your left leg out in front of your chest, left foot planted on the floor pointing forward, and your arms above your head. Lean your body forward until you feel a stretch in the front of your right hip and upper thigh. Hold for 20 seconds. Switch sides.

Note: This can be done with arms down relaxed at your sides.

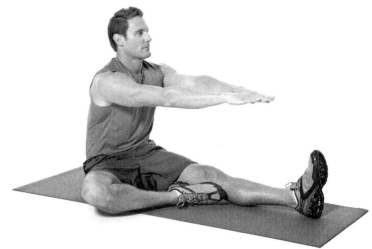

Figure 4 Hamstring Stretch

Sit on the floor in the figure 4 position with your left leg straight out, your foot pointing upward, and your ankle at a 90-degree angle. Sit tall (as if a string were pulling the top of your head toward the ceiling) and reach forward (like a walking zombie), with your index fingers touching side by side. While staying tall and keeping your chest high, slowly lean forward, keeping your left knee straight, and try to touch the wall (at the level of your eyes—i.e., don't reach down toward your toes, but stay tall with good sitting posture). Hold for 20 seconds and then switch sides. Repeat 3 times.

Note: If you are having significant sciatica with leg pain or leg numbness, hold off on the hamstring stretches, especially if they seem to increase leg symptoms. Eventually, as leg symptoms improve, it is important to work on hamstring flexibility.

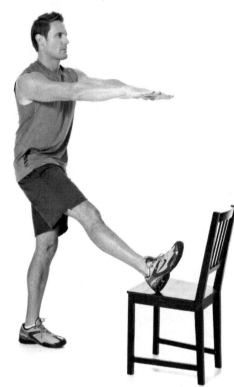

Alternate Hamstring Stretch

Rest your right heel on a chair or low staircase step, keeping your leg perfectly straight. Standing tall with your arms out forward, lean into the chair or staircase as far as you can go and hold for 10 to 20 seconds. Do not lean down and try to touch your toes. Repeat with your left leg.

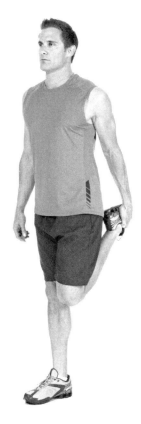

Quad Stretch

Stand upright but use your right hand to support you (until you can balance without difficulty). Grab your left foot with your left hand and bring your heel up to your buttock, keeping your knees together at all times. Stand tall and don't lean forward at the waist or upper body. Hold for 10 seconds and repeat with your right hand and foot.

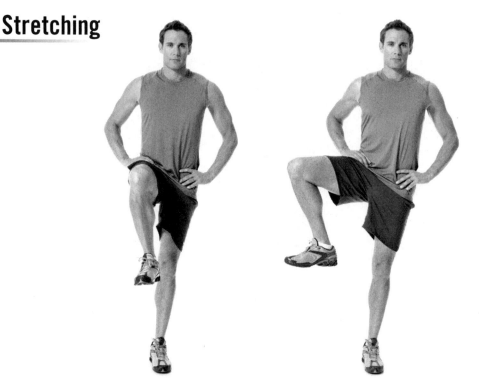

Standing Can Opener

Stand upright, raise your right knee, and flex your hip upward so that it is at 90 degrees, with your thigh approximately at belt height. Tighten your abs as you slowly lift your leg. Keep your abs tight and drawn in as you slowly rotate your right leg as far to the right as it can go, then lower your outwardly turned right foot to the ground so that it forms a "T" with your left foot. Alternate sides. Repeat 3 to 5 times.

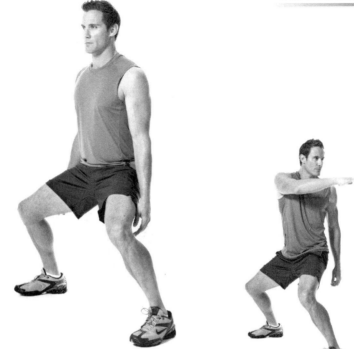

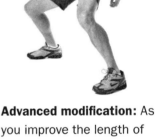

Horse with Ab Hollow

Although the Horse is not really a stretching exercise, done properly it will build leg strength and improve posture. (Anyone with a background in the martial arts will attest to the importance of this one move.) It's a great idea to use the relaxation breathing technique in Step 2 while doing this move.

Start with your feet wider than shoulder-width apart and pointing forward. Stay tall, and keep your back and head straight and your abs tight as you begin to sink into a partial sitting position. Look straight ahead. Keep your knees outward, beyond your feet so that if you look down, your feet are pointing straight ahead on the inner side of your knees. Hold for 20 seconds. Try to build up to a 1-minute hold over subsequent sessions. (If this is too difficult for you, try it while leaning your back flat against a wall. Another alternative is to slowly move up and down from the Horse position to a full standing position, all while concentrating on keeping the abs tight and the pelvis stable.)

Advanced modification: As you improve the length of time holding this position, you can add the side-reach modification, in which you twist your torso area and reach as far as possible to the left side with your right arm, then reach as far as possible to the right side with your left arm, and continue alternating sides.

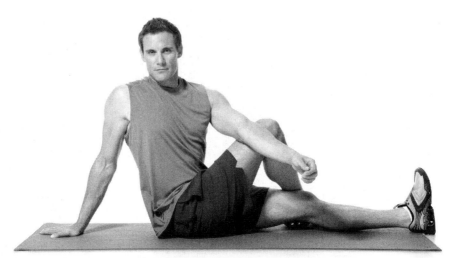

Pretzel ITB

Sit with your left leg straight out and your right foot crossed over and just to the outside of your left knee. Place the outer side of your left elbow on the outer side of your right knee and thigh. Use your left elbow to pull your right knee inward (to the left) and lock it there. You should feel a stretch in the right outer hip and thigh area.

Next, rotate your body so you are looking over your right shoulder as far as you can. (If you are in the center of the room, try to see the left corner behind you.)

Repeat on the opposite side.

■ **KNEE-TO-CHEST (SEE PAGE 103)**

■ **T-ROLL (SEE PAGE 104)**

GO!

You're here at last—the four progressive programs that ensure lower back health for an active life. With one exception that's mentioned later, exercises should be done every other day, or about three times per week—the absolute minimum if your back or body isn't in great shape and you can only tolerate the two lower-intensity levels. After a few weeks of working out regularly, you'll begin to feel better and you'll be able to work harder. Then it won't be long at all before you find yourself doing the advanced program, which usually only has to be done once or twice a week.

You can do your program either as a separate routine or as part of your regular workout regimen at home or at a gym. (Some program exercises require a ball or elastic tubing. If you don't have a gym or rehab facility where this equipment is available, a good ball will only set you back about 30 bucks, and tubing is readily available at minimal cost. Using the Swiss Ball or Thera-Ball, a firm, lightweight ball about the height of a chair—inexpensive and readily available—allows us to build core strength and balance by moderately engaging

all the key torso musculature—abs, obliques, and back. The balls come in different sizes for people of different heights.

5' to 5'6"	55 cm
5'7" to 6'2"	65 cm
6'3" and over	75 cm

I've found the home fitness products at SPRI [www.spri.com] to be first rate. Whatever source you use, be sure to order a ball with the right diameter for your height.) Also, in the Additional Resources section on pages 167–168 is a list of the specific tubing types and door attachments for your home program.

Everyone should start at the beginner level because, regardless of how fit you might be, it's just about a certainty that your lower back frame members have never been worked out like they will be here. If your body doesn't scream at you after three or four sessions, you can move on to the more demanding routines that incorporate additional exercises or increase the intensity of previous ones.

If a particular exercise in a particular program is just not doable for you, but you can handle the others with relative ease, it's perfectly okay to promote yourself to the next level. Once again, use trial and error liberally to find what works for you, and feel free to mix and match exercises from the various levels to customize a program that fits your circumstance.

LEVEL 1: BEGINNER/RECOVERY PROGRAM

If you're not quite over a back episode but you feel you can handle more than the first aid exercises in Step 2, you should use this program often, even daily, until you are able to do it without difficulty.

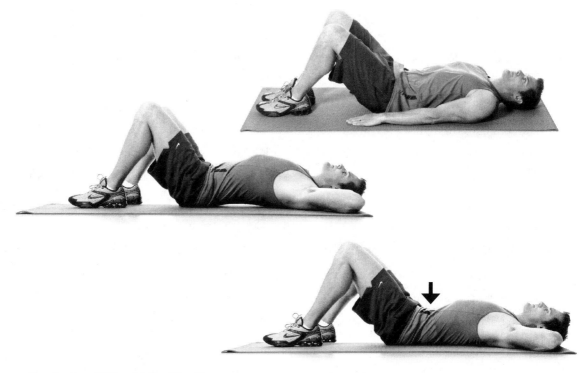

Pelvic Tilt/Ab Hollow

This routine will be the key to any exercise you do, because it teaches you to stabilize your back.

Lie on your back with your knees bent and feet flat on the floor. Pull in your stomach, bringing your belly button toward your spine, tightening your abdominal area. Also gently tighten your gluteal (buttock) muscles. Hold your abdominal area tight, concentrating on a spot approximately 2 inches below your belly button. (You should feel the small of your back flatten toward the floor, reversing the normal curve or arch of your back—but don't try to overflatten your back.) Hold this position for 6 to 10 seconds, then relax. Repeat 5 times.

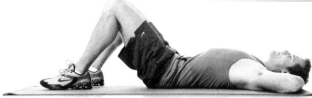

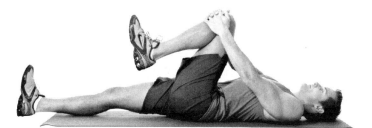

Knee-to-Chest

Start with the Pelvic Tilt and hold. Pull your left leg/knee toward your chest with your hands behind the knee area (or in front if that is more comfortable). Breathe gently and relax, keeping your head on the floor. Hold for 10 to 20 seconds, then repeat with the right leg.

Next, pull both knees to your chest. Relax and hold for 10 to 20 seconds. (If you are comfortable with these static positions, you can add a slight rocking motion.)

Repeat this sequence 3 to 4 times.

Level 1: Beginner/Recovery Program

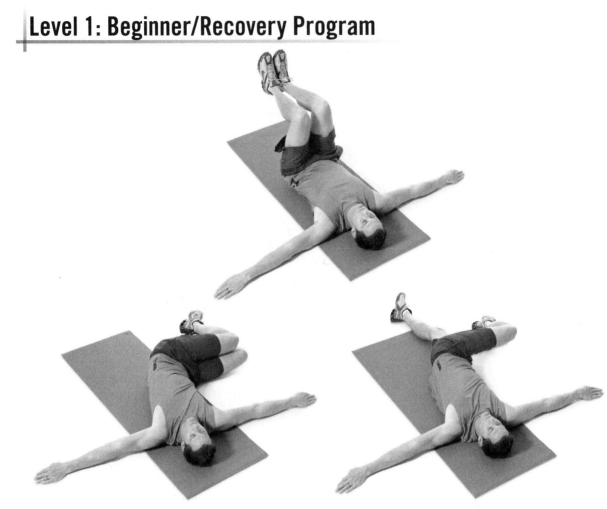

T-Roll

Lie on your back with your legs straight and your arms stretched out so that you form a T. Bring both of your knees up so that your hips and knees are flexed to 90 degrees. Keeping your palms, elbows, and shoulders on the floor (don't let them lift off), twist your torso and rotate your pelvis and knees so that your right knee is on the floor by your side (keeping your knees together). Hold for 5 to 7 seconds. Repeat on the opposite side. Repeat this sequence 2 times.

Alternate T-Roll: Keep your right leg straight while rotating your left leg over to the floor at your right. Repeat on the opposite side as with T-Roll.

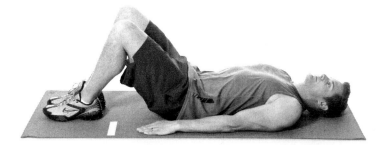

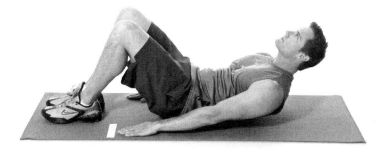

Pre-Crunch (Curlup)

Lie on your back with your arms at your sides, palms down, your knees bent to 90 degrees, and both feet resting on the floor (keeping legs bent help protect your lower back). Tighten your abs, and slowly lift your head and shoulders slightly off the floor while allowing your hands to slide along the floor approximately 6 to 8 inches (see hand position in second photo with tape on mat). Do not flex or strain your neck or tuck your chin. Hold for 8 seconds and repeat 10 times.

Note: If this movement is too uncomfortable, try it with your right foot on the floor and your left leg crossed with your left ankle resting on your right knee. Do the curlups and then switch legs.

Level 1: Beginner/Recovery Program

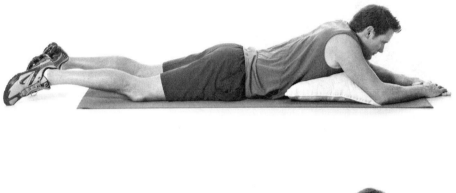

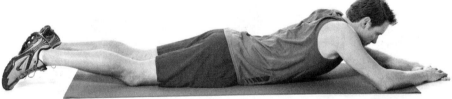

Pre-Cobra

Lie on your stomach on the floor or on a mat with one or two pillows under your chest to create a gentle arch in your back. Hold for 2 to 3 minutes.

You can also try this without a pillow, supporting yourself slightly upward with your arms out in front as shown in lower photo.

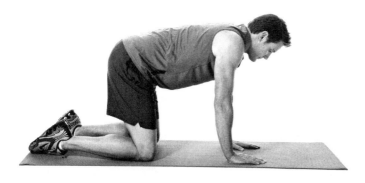

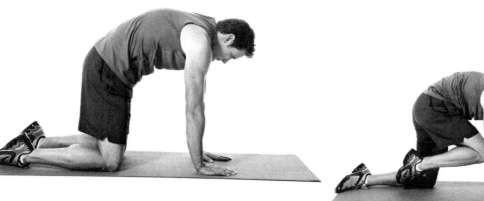

Cat

Kneel on the floor and support your weight on your palms in front of you, keeping your arms straight and your back flat. Your knees should be under your hips. Looking down, keep your neck relaxed and inhale, slowly pulling in your stomach. At the same time, arch your back upward as if a string were attached to your mid-back area, pulling it upward like a cat. Hold for 5 seconds and repeat twice.

Cat modification: Do the Cat as described, while spine is still straight (as in first photo) and parallel to the floor, tighten your abs and slowly pull your right knee up toward your chest, hold 3 to 5 seconds and then lower it. Repeat with left leg. Do 5 reps with each.

Level 1: Beginner/Recovery Program

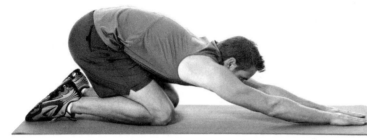

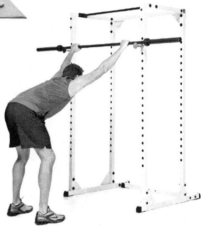

Child's Pose

After completing the Cat, rise back to a kneeling position. Gently sit back onto your heels (or as far as you can comfortably go). Lower your forehead and chest area toward the floor as your arms (palms down) reach forward. Slide your palms forward as far as they will go, feeling both a relaxation and stretch in the spine, latissimus, and shoulder area. Hold for 5 seconds.

Standing modification: Lean forward along a Smith machine, barbell rack, or countertop with your arms straight out while bending at the waist and looking downward. Gently rock your hips and pelvis backward until you feel a stretch in the upper back, lat, and shoulder area.

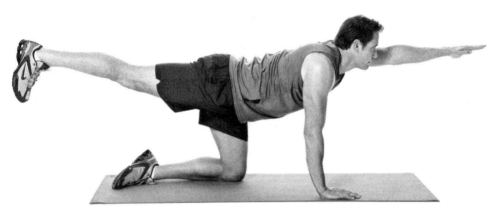

Bird Dog

Start on the floor on all fours. Slowly lift your left arm and right leg simultaneously, holding both straight for 5 to 7 seconds. Do not raise your arm or leg above horizontal; instead, stay parallel to the ground. Alternate sides and do 5 reps on each side.

Modified Bird Dog: If the full Bird Dog is too difficult, or if you have significant discomfort, try raising only one arm or one leg at a time, and gradually build up to where you can hold both out, even if they are only partially held out rather than fully.

Advanced Bird Dog: Using ankle weights and a small hand weight, add 3 to 5 pounds per limb.

Level 1: Beginner/Recovery Program

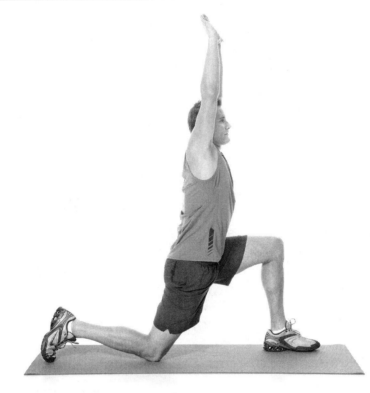

Psoas Stretch (kneeling)

As I stated in Step 1, you've got to work the iliopsoas muscle to relieve hip and back pain.

Kneel on your right knee with your left leg out in front of your chest, and your left foot planted on the floor and pointing forward. Raise both arms over your head with palms together. Lean your body forward until you feel a stretch in the front of your right hip and upper thigh. Hold for 20 seconds, then switch sides.

Note: This stretch can also be done with arms relaxed at your sides. The arms-up version gives a better stretch and improves posture. Keep hands over head, palms together. Reach as high as you can and stay tall with a straight spine.

LEVEL 2:
INTERMEDIATE PROGRAM

If you're in decent physical condition and your lower back is behaving, but you haven't exercised strenuously on a regular basis in the recent past, this level will probably suit you best (for a short time, however, because you're implementing the comprehensive fitness recommendations in this book, right?). It's at this

level that you'll discover just how good your back can feel, and you'll start to see a lot more possibility for activities you might not have done in a while. (Directions and photos for the first 3 and 6th exercises are in Step 2.)

- **PELVIC TILT/AB HOLLOW (SEE PAGE 102)**
- **KNEE-TO-CHEST (SEE PAGE 103)**
- **T-ROLL (SEE PAGE 104)**

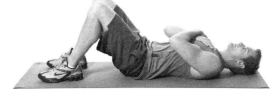

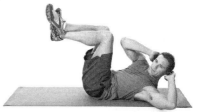

Crunch

Start with a Pelvic Tilt, tightening abs, knees bent, feet resting on the floor. Do not throw yourself forward. Do not clasp your hands behind your head, but keep them near your ears or across your chest. Do not anchor your feet under anything or have someone hold your feet, as this allows you to use your hip flexor muscles rather than your abs. Tighten your abdominal muscles and slowly curl your head and shoulders off the floor; feel your breastbone accordion in toward your upper pubic bone. Don't use your hands to pull your neck or head forward, and keep your lower back on the floor. Pause momentarily; then, very slowly, in a controlled manner, come back down. Slowly exhale during the lifting phase and inhale during the lowering phase. Do 20 repetitions.

Note: In most gyms, there are great machine options for total abdominal work, and they include the ab machines or machine crunch as well as the rotary torso for obliques. There are also numerous alternatives that are worth incorporating into your workouts at various times. The basic crunch tends to work the upper abdominal area. To target your lower abdominal area, do a hanging knee raise from a chinup bar or do a reverse crunch.

Advanced modification— Crunch with a Twist: Lie on your back with your ankles crossed and your hips and knees flexed at 90-degree angles. Slowly perform a crunch, bringing your right elbow to your left knee. Hold for 3 seconds. Do 10 repetitions and repeat on the opposite side. Or, for a slightly easier version, lie on your back with your right knee bent and foot resting on the floor. Cross your left leg over your right knee. Keep your left arm out on the floor. Place your right hand near your right ear and slowly twist up, bringing your right elbow toward your left knee.

Level 2: Intermediate Program

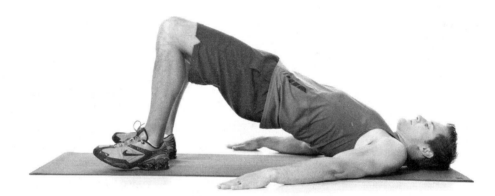

Glute Bridge

Lie on the floor with your knees bent to 90 degrees, your feet flat on the floor hip-width apart, and your arms resting on the floor to support you. Tighten your abs and lift or bridge your hips toward the ceiling while tightening your glutes (buttock muscles). Hold for 3 to 5 seconds and then lower your torso without letting your buttocks touch the floor. You should feel this in your glutes and not your hamstrings or lower back. Repeat 5 to 7 times.

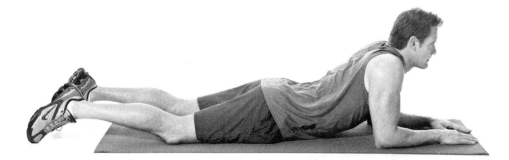

Mid-Cobra

Lie on your stomach. Slowly extend your back by propping yourself up onto your elbows. Always keep the front of your hips and pelvis on the floor; don't let them lift off. Keep your neck in a comfortable position, especially if you have neck problems; don't look up. Hold for 20 to 30 seconds. Repeat twice.

Level 2: Intermediate Program

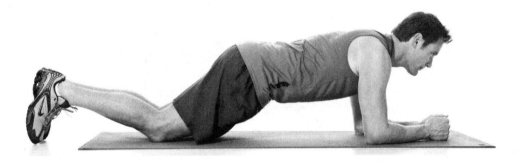

Front Plank (kneeling)

Lie on your stomach with your forearms and elbows resting on the floor. Keeping your knees on the floor, tighten your abs and lift your chest and pelvis off the floor with your forearms supporting your weight. Keep your back straight. Hold for 20 to 30 seconds. Repeat twice.

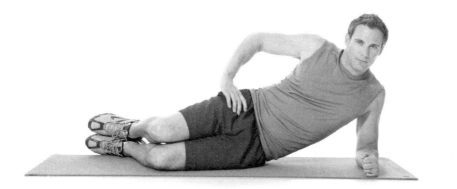

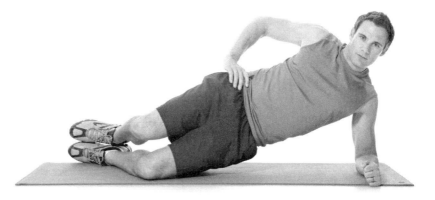

Side Plank (on knees)

Lie on your left side with your left forearm and elbow on the floor. Your elbow should be in line with your shoulder, and your torso sagging toward the floor. Lean into your forearm, lifting your hips in the air to form a straight, rigid line while supporting your weight on your forearm and knees. Hold for 20 seconds. Repeat twice and then perform again lying on your right side.

Advanced Side Plank: Try to increase your hold time to 1 to 2 minutes. If this gets too easy, hold a light weight against the hip that's on top.

Level 2: Intermediate Program

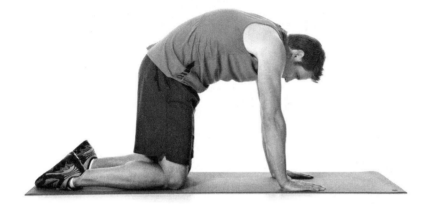

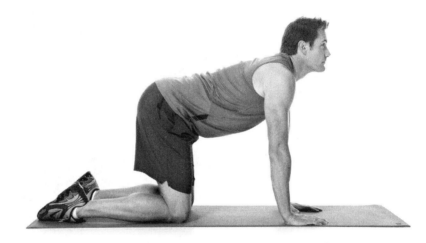

Dynamic Cat/Cow

This flexion/extension cycle can improve spinal mobility and enhance nourishment to the deeper spinal structures. It is a gentle dynamic motion exercise and not a stretch, so don't push the extremes of motion. The emphasis should be on a rocking motion rather than extreme stretching.

Start on all fours. Arch your back upward, performing a Cat movement (described on page 107). Next, relax your spine so that it sags downward. Repeat 5 to 7 cycles.

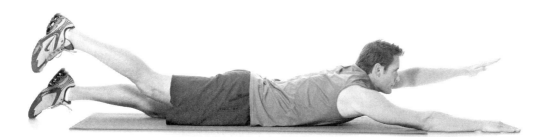

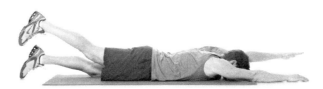

Partial Superman

Lie facedown on the floor with your arms straight out in line with your legs (picture Superman flying in the air). Raise your left arm and right leg off the floor. Keep your knee straight so that your leg is being lifted by your buttocks and lower back. If it does not bother your neck, your head should also come off the floor. Hold for 10 seconds and build up to 20 seconds. Repeat with your right arm and left leg. Do 5 reps on each side.

Modifications: If you have neck problems, you can keep your face resting on the floor and not lift your head. If you are unable to do even the beginner version, you can start with just lifting only one arm or leg off the floor and build up as tolerated.

LEVEL 3: ADVANCED PROGRAM

Those who make physical fitness a priority, who work out and play hard, will find these exercises particularly useful and should reach this level after 2 to 4 weeks. Regardless of when it is reached, it is a terrific preventive maintenance program for the lower back. Many individuals are content to stop at this level, especially if they do not have high-demand bodies.

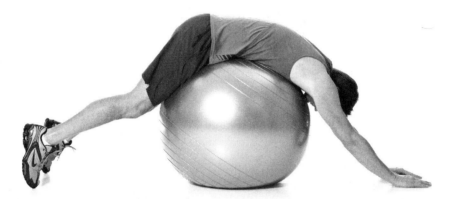

Spinal Stretch/Drape on Ball

This is a terrific lower back relaxation technique that I use very often on its own. It will stretch the entire spine (especially the lower back) and buttock and hamstring areas, and it will help reverse lumbar lordosis (tightness of the lower back often causing the lower back to arch).

Lie facedown on the ball with your toes touching the floor and your arms stretched out in front, reaching forward. Let your spine and entire body relax. Perform Relaxation Breathing from Level 2, page 79. Hold for 20 to 30 seconds or as long as you like if you find this comfortable.

Modifications: If this position is uncomfortable, start with the Drape, which is a "tighter" version of this exercise with your hands and feet closer to the ball. You can even start by kneeling on the floor, hugging the ball. Progress to where your knees are off the floor but remain slightly flexed and closer to the ball. As flexibility, stability, and balance improve, you can progress to the full Spinal Stretch.

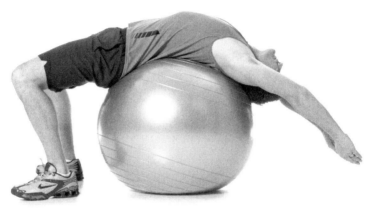

Spinal Extension (passive stretch)/ Passive Extension on Ball

This will stretch and relax the entire spine and is excellent for posture, especially for people who tend to hunch forward or who have thoracic kyphosis, in which the mid- to upper spine is flexed forward.

Start by sitting on the ball with your feet on the floor. Slowly step forward, letting the ball roll backward to your lower back area so that your back arches backward over the ball. Lie back, initially keeping your arms crossed on your chest. Next reach backward, opening up your shoulders, and try to reach toward the floor behind you. Hold for 10 to 20 seconds. Repeat twice.

Modifications: You can slightly roll back and forth to improve the stretch and massage your spinal area. As you improve your spinal mobility, you can advance to where your hands reach back to touch the floor.

Level 3: Advanced Program

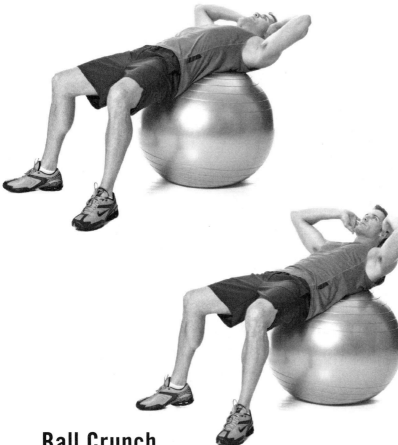

Ball Crunch

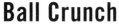

Lie on the ball with your hands behind your ears or across your chest and your feet resting on the floor. Tighten and hollow your abs and slowly curl up, concentrating on using your abs so that your head and shoulders come up to a position that is approximately halfway between lying and sitting. Hold for 5 seconds. Roll back slowly to the starting position, keeping your abs tight all the way back. Repeat 20 times. (An advanced version is to start from a position farther back over the ball, i.e., step backward and let the ball roll forward slightly under you.)

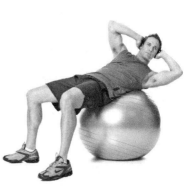

Ball Crunch with Twist: Do the crunch as described, but as you slowly curl up, rotate at your waist, alternating left and right before you reach the halfway position. Repeat 20 times on each side.

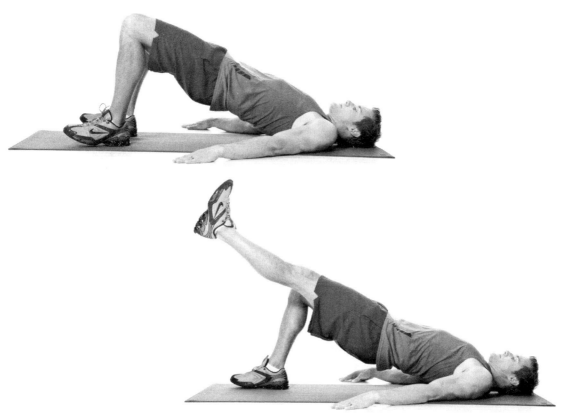

Glute Bridge (with leg up)

Lie on the floor with your knees bent to 90 degrees, your feet flat on the floor hip-width apart, and your arms away from your body (at 45-degree angles) and resting on the floor to support you. Tighten your abs and lift or bridge your hips toward the ceiling while tightening your glutes (buttock muscles). Next, slowly extend your left leg so that it is straight out, toes pointing toward the ceiling. Hold your left leg out for 5 seconds and then lower it, maintaining the firm bridge position at all times throughout this exercise until all reps are completed. Next, repeat with your right leg. Complete 10 repetitions with each leg.

Level 3: Advanced Program

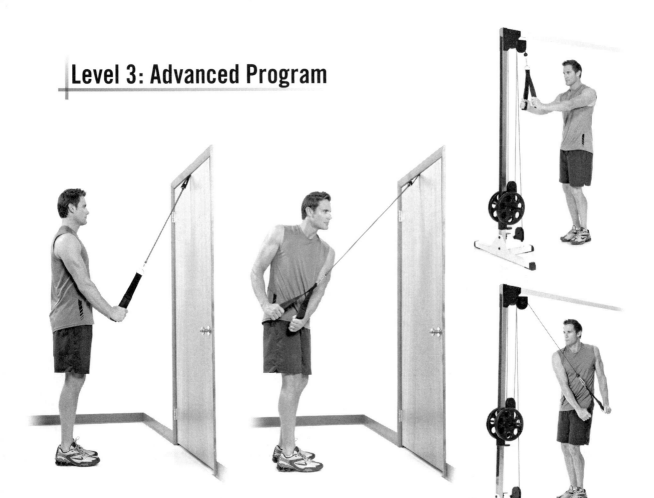

Twist-O

Using a machine pulley system, stand with your feet slightly wider than your shoulders. Hold the handles in front of you with your arms out and elbows slightly bent. Tighten and hollow your abdominal area. Now, using your abdominal and torso area (not arms or lats), rotate your midsection and slowly bring your left hand down toward the outer side of your right hip or thigh. Pause for 3 seconds, keeping your abdominal area tucked in and tightened. Keep your shoulders and chest facing mostly forward to better isolate and activate your abdominal core muscles. Return to the starting position and repeat on the opposite side. Do 10 reps on each side.

Modification: This is a terrific exercise to do on a cable-type machine at the gym, where increased weights can be added as you get stronger. If it's done correctly, focusing mentally on the abdominal area and torso (and not the arms or upper body) to perform the movement, not much weight or resistance is needed.

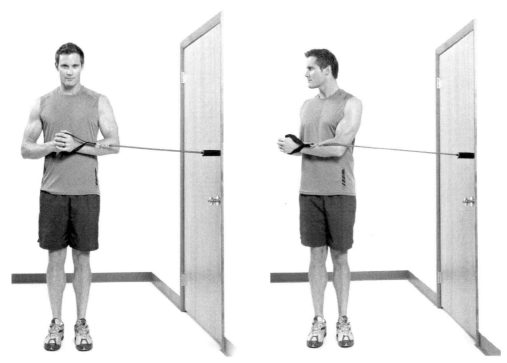

Spinal Rotation (with tubing)

Using tubing firmly attached (at elbow height) to a door frame, stand with your left side facing the door and your feet slightly wider than your shoulders. Begin by holding the tubing with both hands toward your left side. Tighten your abs and, using your torso and abdominal muscles, rotate toward your right side, using the tubing as resistance. Start with a tension that allows 20 reps. Repeat on the opposite side. As this gets easier, increase the resistance by either re-tensioning/tightening the tubing or using tubing that offers greater resistance.

Note: This can also be done on an adjustable cable machine.

Level 3: Advanced Program

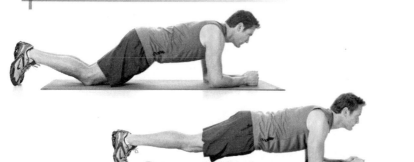

Quadruped

While kneeling on the floor, place your forearms flat on the floor as if you were to do a modified pushup. Now, assume the plank position with your body straight and your full weight supported on both forearms and your toes (second photo). Your body should be straight as a board with your pelvis tucked inward, tightening your abdominal and buttock muscles. Try holding that position with your weight on your forearms and toes for 60 seconds.

Next, lift your right arm off the floor for 15 seconds, supporting your full weight on your left arm and both feet (third photo). Repeat, lifting your left arm.

With both forearms on the floor, raise your right leg, hold for 15 seconds, and then repeat, lifting your left leg.

Next, try to elevate your right arm and left leg simultaneously (fourth photo) and hold for 15 seconds, then return them to the floor and repeat with your left arm and right leg raised.

Return to the plank position and hold for 30 seconds.

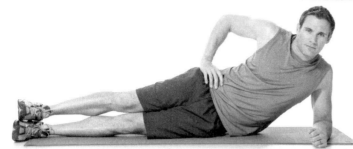

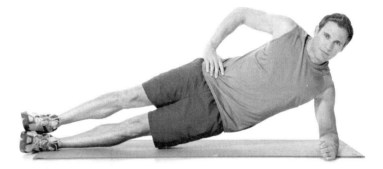

Side Plank (full)

Lie on your left side, with your left forearm and elbow on the floor. Your elbow should be in line with your shoulder, and your torso sagging toward the floor. Lean on your forearm, lifting your hips and knees upward into a straight, rigid line while supporting all your weight on your forearm and the side of your left foot. Hold for 20 seconds. Repeat twice and then perform the exercise again, lying on your right side.

Alternate version: Instead of stacking one foot directly on the other, try performing this plank with the foot of the top leg also resting on the floor just in front of your other foot.

Advanced Side Plank: Try to increase your hold time to 1 to 2 minutes. If this gets too easy, hold a light weight against the hip that's on top.

Level 3: Advanced Program

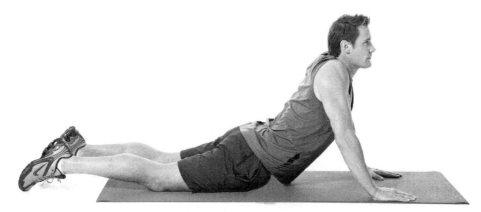

Cobra

Lie on your stomach. Raise yourself, keeping your hips and pelvis on the floor, until your upper body is supported by your palms with your arms almost fully extended (just shy of elbow lockout position). Hold for 30 seconds. Repeat twice.

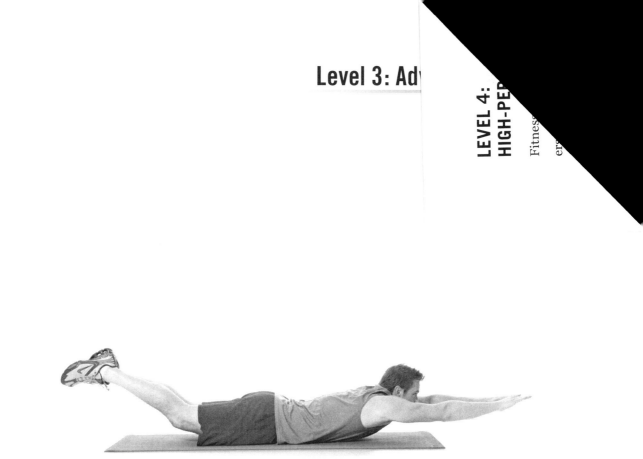

Superman

I first described this exercise almost 30 years ago both to assess spinal muscle strength and to help individuals rebuild their lower backs after injury. This exercise is terrific for spinal extensor muscle strength and maintaining overall spine health.

Lie on the floor facedown with your arms straight out, in line with your legs. (Picture Superman flying in the air.) Simultaneously bring both arms and both legs off the floor. Only your abdominal area and pelvis should be touching the floor. Hold for 10 seconds and build up to 20 seconds. Do 10 reps.

RFORMANCE PROGRAM

fanatics, dancers and other perform-
, and top athletes (including professionals)
should aspire to this level of physical exercise.
It will not only protect your spine, keeping it
healthy and less vulnerable, but will also
improve performance. Using a gym ball for
this entire program is what makes it the most
challenging, because the most frame members (bones and connective tissues) are
engaged as you do each routine. Check the
Additional Resources at the end of the book
for the specific types of tubing and door
attachments needed for these exercises.

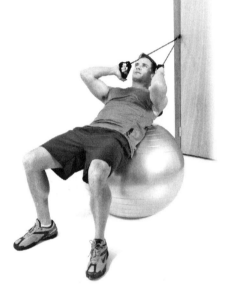

Ball Crunch with Tubing/Resistance

Using tubing firmly attached to a door frame (approximately at
chest height), lie on the ball with your back toward the door
and the tubing across your shoulders, held by your hands near
your chest. Tighten your abs and slowly curl up, concentrating
on using your abs so that your head and shoulders come up to
a position that is approximately halfway between lying and sitting. Hold for 5 seconds, then roll back slowly to the starting
position, keeping your abs tight all the way back. Start with a
tension that allows 20 reps. As this gets easier, increase the
resistance by re-tensioning/tightening the tubing, or using tubing that offers greater resistance.

**Alternate Ball Crunch
with Resistance:** Instead
of tubing, use a light
weight (5-pound plate or
dumbbell) held behind your
head for resistance.

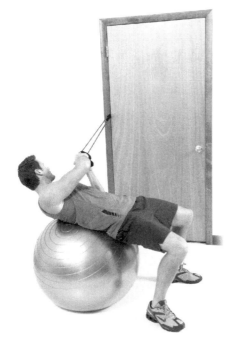
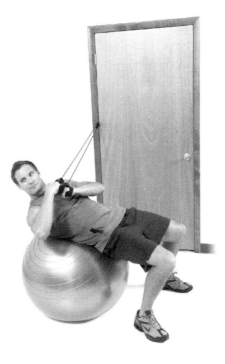

Crunch Twist on Ball with Tubing/Resistance

Using tubing firmly attached to a door frame, lie on the ball with your left side toward the door and the tubing tensioned over your left shoulder. While holding the crunch and tightening your abs, rotate at your waist, twisting toward the right using your obliques. Repeat 20 times, then switch to the opposite side.

Alternate Crunch Twist on Ball with Resistance:
Instead of tubing, use a light weight, such as a 5-pound plate or dumbbell, held behind your head for resistance.

Level 4: High-Performance Program

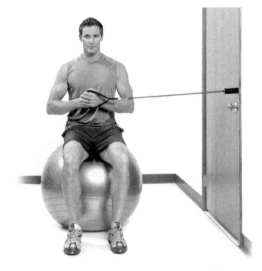 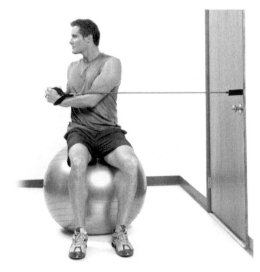

Spinal Rotation on Ball with Tubing/Resistance

Using tubing firmly attached to a door frame (at waist height when standing), sit on a ball with your left side facing the door. Begin by holding the tubing with both hands toward your left side. Tighten your abs and, using your torso and abdominal muscles, rotate toward your right side using the tubing as resistance. Start with a tension that allows 20 reps. Repeat on the opposite side. As this gets easier, increase the resistance by either re-tensioning/tightening the tubing or using tubing that offers greater resistance.

Alternate Spinal Rotation with Medicine Ball: Holding a small weighted medicine ball in your hands, recline on the gym ball, slightly forward so that your lower back is fully supported. Tighten your abs and slowly sit up into the crunch position while twisting to your right with the medicine ball held out just outside your right thigh. While maintaining the crunch, twist to the left thigh area. Do 10 reps to each side. Move in a slow, controlled fashion, rather than rapid fire.

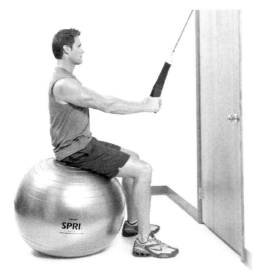 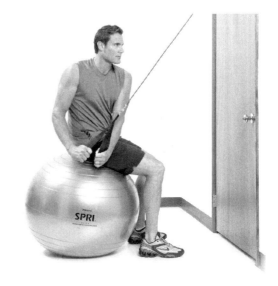

Twist-O (seated) on Ball with Tubing/Resistance

Using tubing firmly attached to the upper part of a door frame, sit on a ball facing the door. Hold the tubing with both hands in front of you. Tighten your abdominal area. Using your abdominal and torso areas (not arms or lats), rotate your midsection and slowly bring both hands down toward the outer side of your right hip or thigh, pausing for 3 seconds and keeping your abdominal area tucked in and tightened. Return to the starting position and repeat on the opposite side. Do 10 reps on each side. As this gets easier, increase the resistance by either re-tensioning/tightening the tubing or using tubing that offers greater resistance.

Modification: Many gyms or home gyms have an upper cable attachment that allows this exact motion to be done with weights.

Level 4: High-Performance Program

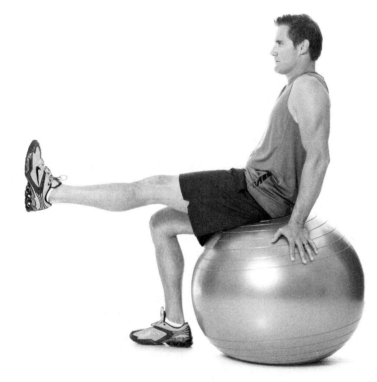

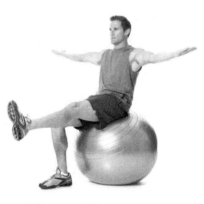

Seated Leg Extension on Ball

This will improve balance; core, quadriceps, and hamstring strength; and hamstring flexibility. Sit on the ball, tall and upright, with your feet no more than shoulder-width apart and your hands resting on the sides of the ball. Tighten your abdominal muscles. Keeping your right foot flat on the floor, extend your left leg fully, tightening your thigh muscles. Hold for 10 seconds. Repeat 5 times with each leg.

Advanced: Remove your hands from the ball and keep them out to the sides so your body forms a T. For even more of a challenge, add ankle weights. Start with 1 or 2 pounds. Also try doing this while on the ball of your foot, rather than keeping your foot flat on the floor.

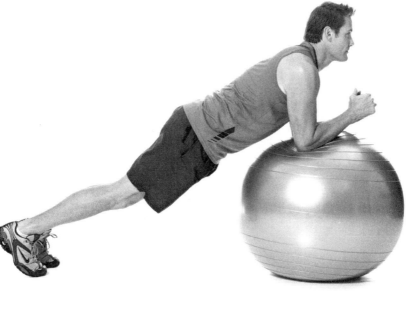

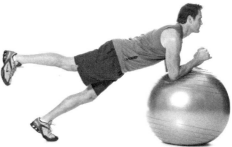

Bridge/Plank on Ball

Kneel facing a ball, resting your elbows and forearms on the ball. Tighten your abs and lift upward into the Plank position so that your back and legs form a straight line and you are supported only on your elbows and feet. Hold for 20 seconds, keeping your abs and torso area tightened and stabilized, and repeat twice. Try to build up to 1 minute.

Advanced: **Perform the Plank on the ball as described, and once you are stabilized and secure, slowly lift your right leg in a straight line using your gluteal (buttock) muscles.** Hold for 20 seconds and then change legs. Repeat twice with each leg.

Level 4: High-Performance Program

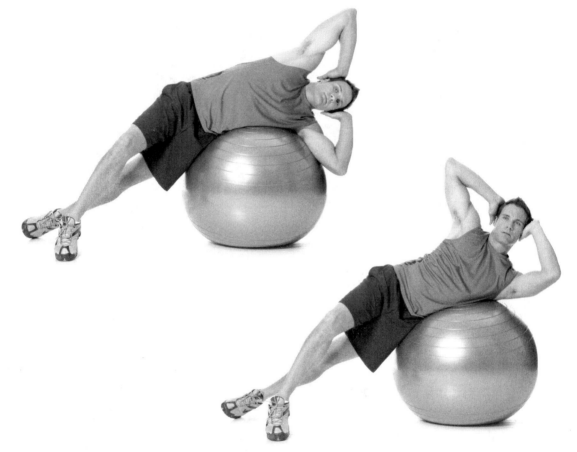

Trunk Side Bend on Ball

Lie on your side on the ball with your arms up and your hands by your head. Cross your legs to create a stable base with both feet on the floor and your legs straight. The top leg will be in front of your body and the bottom leg behind it. Tighten your abs and slowly lift your body upward to form a straight line. Hold for 3 seconds and slowly let yourself back down. Repeat 10 times on each side.

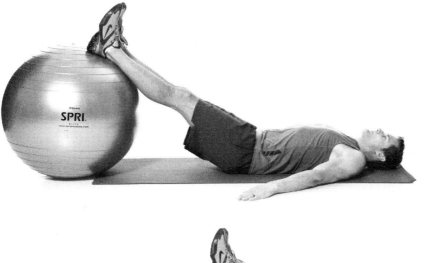

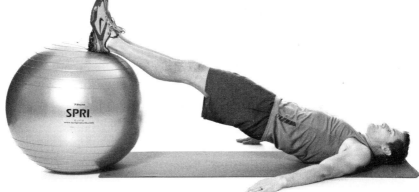

Glute Bridge on Ball

Lie on the floor with your heels on the ball and toes pointing upward, arms and palms resting flat on the floor slightly away from your body. Tighten your glutes (buttock muscles), lifting your pelvis upward to form a straight line. Only your head, shoulders, and arms will be on the floor. Hold for 3 seconds and slowly drop back down to the floor. Repeat 5 times.

Advanced: Try the Glute Bridge on the ball, but this time cross your arms in front of your chest, making balance more difficult.

Level 4: High-Performance Program

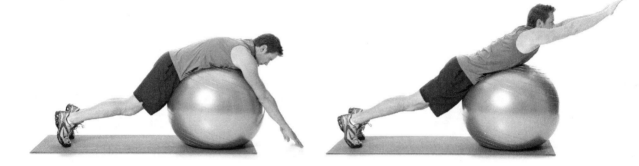

Superman on Ball (active spinal extension)

This exercise is for spinal extensor muscle strength and endurance and gluteal strength. From the Spinal Stretch position on the ball (see page 118), keeping your feet on the floor and your legs straight, slowly extend your lumbar area until you are straight or slightly extended in the lower back area and your arms are fully extended beyond your head, like Superman flying. Hold for 10 seconds and build up to 20 seconds. Do 5 to 10 repetitions.

More advanced alternative: Get into the Superman position and then gently lift one straight leg off the floor, balancing only on the opposite straightened leg. This further strengthens the gluteal area. Hold for 5 seconds, then alternate legs.

Most advanced version: Do the full Superman, in which only your abdominal area is on the ball and both feet and arms are outward in the "flying" position. Feet should be off the floor.

Modified version: If you are unable to perform the exercises listed above, start by assisting yourself, keeping your hands on the floor and just slightly lifting them off the floor when possible. Gradually build up to where you can straighten your back fully and then start bringing your hands upward to the full Superman.

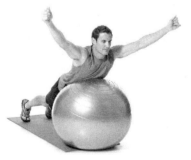

Note: Another Superman alternative that also helps with shoulder and upper back strength involves performing the basic Superman exercise, with your feet on the floor, but instead of your arms reaching straight out forward like Superman's, they can be placed either in a Y or T formation. Keep your thumbs pointing up when using the Y or T version.

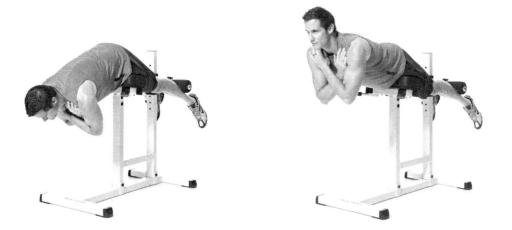

Roman chair version: You can also improve spinal extension strength using a Roman chair. This exercise does not isolate the lumbar muscles as well, because the gluteus muscles and upper hamstrings help with the movement. Also, because the ball is not used, less overall spinal stability is achieved. Hook your feet under the leg anchors on the chair. Fold arms across your chest and raise torso until it's in line with your legs. Hold for 20 seconds. Do 5 to 10 repetitions.

As noted throughout this book, spinal extensor strength is one of the cornerstones of lower back pain prevention and treatment. For those who are having ongoing issues, I strongly recommend finding a gym or physical therapy facility that offers isolated spinal strengthening equipment, such as the MedX lumbar extension machine. MedX offers both testing and strengthening/rehabilitation equipment and is invaluable for those with chronic lower back pain.

"BACK" TO THE FUTURE

Whether you define "active" as being able to play competitive singles tennis or as being able to move about and perform your usual daily tasks, you'll be "active for life" if you commit to a regular workout program. The specifics and level of your physical fitness are unique to you, but *action* is something that applies to every case.

Hurting or not, your frame requires attention if it is to recover from injury and stay healthy. What you are able to do to support it isn't critical; doing *something* is. The whole idea is to do the appropriate targeted exercises, the ones you can tolerate, and progress at your own pace. Remember, this is not a competition.

Use the ones that work best for you more often, and avoid those that cause significant discomfort (but don't forget to try them again later when your back improves). Over time, and with some trial and error, you will probably develop your own optimal routine, as this is not a "one size fits all" program. It sometimes takes a little detective work to determine which exercises are best for your situation and which should be avoided. If you are having difficulty advancing, try adding only one new exercise per session to see how you tolerate it. Sometimes an exercise feels good while you are doing it, but later that evening, or the next day, you are in trouble. If you've added numerous exercises, it becomes difficult to determine which one or two were the culprits. You might have to stay at a low level of exercise indefinitely, or you might wind up going back and forth between levels, but that's okay. As long as you keep taking steps, however small, you'll be in far better shape down the road.

BACK TALK

If you have to take this step, your back issues are very serious. Although the facts are that 80 percent of aching backs are better in 2 weeks, another 10 percent are better by week 4, and most are much better after another month has gone by, that still leaves a small percentage whose back pain is chronic and doesn't respond to the first aid remedies in Step 2. If you're among them, the full program in the previous step is simply out of the question.

Temporarily, however.

Because there's still a lot you can do to restore your frame.

If you have an ailing back that seems to be your constant companion or afflicts you without much respite in between, and you are not a candidate for surgical intervention, pay close attention to the remedial approaches in the coming pages. (And if you aren't in this category of people who suffer from back pain, by no means should you skip this step—there are some kernels that will make self-management of your back issues more effective and will help keep future episodes at bay. At the very

least, armed with this knowledge, you might just be able to really help someone else.)

Take heart: Relief is at hand. It's available from a host of caring, skilled people who provide professional help, but it still starts with you. You're the one who is seeking a path out of the wilderness, and finding it requires due diligence on your part: educating yourself about everything that's available, trying the approaches that appeal most to you, and sticking to the ones that work in your circumstances.

But before we get to the good stuff, a brief reminder and a critical warning are in store.

BACK STORY

I'll admit that pain is tricky. But if your case is closely supervised and no additional harm will be caused, suck it up and find out exactly what activities you are able to do. People say, "I'm hurt, I can't work." I ask: If it hurts at home, wouldn't it hurt pretty much the same way if you were sitting at a desk doing some work, answering a phone, being productive?

GOOD BACKS—AND BAD ONES— ARE A MATTER OF HABIT

A solid foundation is the basis for lasting recovery from a chronically out-of-whack back. You build one by maintaining the best behaviors we discussed earlier.

■ QUIT SMOKING

We could never say this too much. Nicotine, in all of its forms, blocks the transport of oxygen and vital nutrients to disks and the rest of your spine members. This causes them to decline faster, hinders self-repair, and delays—or eliminates—recovery from surgery.

■ GET THOSE EXTRA POUNDS OFF YOUR FRAME

Taxing your body with extra weight is a prescription for trouble when you're otherwise healthy. Doing so when you're trying to get your back quieted down is a handicap that in and of itself could compromise all of your efforts.

■ STRIVE FOR PERFECT POSTURE

Slouched shoulders, a drooping head, and locked knees place enormous stress on the spine. When seated, support your lumbar area, keep your shoulders back, and tuck your chin in slightly.

Remember, some of the highest forces on your lower back occur in the seated position, especially if you slouch a little. Riding in cars can be a real challenge, but newer car seats have lumbar supports that can be adjusted, or you can invest in a small lumbar support. Also, take frequent breaks on longer trips to get out, move about, and nourish your spine. When standing and walking, keep your feet slightly apart, your knees straight (but not locked out), and your shoulders and chin under control as they are when you're sitting. And, ladies, shoes can be problematic; the higher the heel, the more your back must arch to compensate, creating postural issues that your lower back does not appreciate in its effort to stay healthy.

WATCH THOSE BLTs!

Whether you're picking up something heavy or just a feather, get close to the object, bend your knees, grasp the object firmly, lift straight up *without twisting*, hold the object close to your body, move close to where you want to place the object, and bend your knees when lowering it, even if that's just a short distance.

EXERCISE

Chronic back pain being what it is, it's likely that something is throbbing or barking whether you're in motion or at rest. Believe me—I know that it can take over your thoughts and your decisions about what you are going to do. But don't let it imprison you. Instead, try to distract yourself, fool your mind in some way so you'll keep trying those recovery routines in Step 2. Believe me when I say that a breakthrough is just around the corner.

CHECK YOUR VITAMIN D LEVEL

A peer-reviewed examination of 22 research studies revealed that almost all patients with chronic back pain had inadequate levels of vitamin D, and, more important, there was plenty of evidence that proper supplementation (1,000 IU of vitamin D and 2,000 IU of vitamin D_3 daily) can provide relief.

One study involving 360 patients who had been given vitamin D over 3 months revealed that the pain either vanished or was helped to a significant extent in 95 percent of the cases. (This is not to say that vitamin D is a miracle cure. It is, however, an important factor that might be overlooked in chronic back pain cases and might, indeed, help in an overall program for back recovery.)

MAINTAIN A HEALTHY MIND FRAME

Prolonged distress and pain take a toll on you and affect your entire outlook on life. You are human, after all. There's no shame in that, but you must not let your ongoing travails take you to a place where recovery is severely compromised or precluded altogether. Revisit the extensive chilling-out

BACKBOARD

approaches in Step 4 on a regular basis—every day, if need be.

You've simply got to be aware of how your mind affects frame recovery and health. If you're stressed out, anxious, or depressed, tell your doctor. And if he or she glosses over this critical aspect of your case and is only interested in the remedies of his or her specialty, don't give in. Treat your mind, and it'll be a heck of lot easier, and more effective, when your body gets treated.

MEDICATION ABUSE

An FDA advisory group has recently urged a ban on Vicodin and Percocet, and strongly rec-

ommends drastic changes in the way people use the popular painkillers acetaminophen and ibuprofen. It cautions that even when these latter two over-the-counter products are used as their labels recommend, overdosing may occur and cause liver damage or gastrointestinal bleeding—*and it might even be fatal!* Likewise, steroids have substantial gastrointestinal risks, and extended use of them can lead to osteopenia, serious infection, osteonecrosis (death of bone tissue), and a variety of other problems.

Most spine specialists know that the best painkillers can be counterproductive when managing lower back pain, especially when it is chronic. Narcotics like OxyContin, Percocet, and codeine do help with more serious pain, but they are highly addictive and don't really help resolve the root source of the pain. It's very tempting to try to soothe your aches with narcotics, but in the long run you'll just be adding an addiction to your ongoing backache.

You will never get rid of a pain problem if you have an addiction going on.

For severe acute back pain, I'd reluctantly recommend a few days of narcotics for select patients. I'm not being mean or insensitive,

BACK STORY

I've had my share of significant "back attacks," but I have never taken a narcotic or sedative. I'm not being stoic, just smart. Painkillers don't solve the problem, and they could hamper progress toward full recovery. They could lead to serious addiction, and they can even be lethal. A recent study of 2,400 patients who had had lumbar fusion surgery linked narcotics to one in five of the 103 deaths that occurred within 3 years of the procedure. Whether you're a candidate for surgery or not, narcotics are dangerous, no matter when you take them. Both you and your doctor must use extreme caution to ensure any pain medication is properly used.

because I, along with many other doctors, feel you will never get rid of a pain problem if you have an addiction going on. The easiest thing for a patient to do is to ask for a pain medication prescription, and the easiest thing for a physician to do is to write one (or a couple). But if I'm really putting the patient's best interests first, I'll take the time to explain why narcotics aren't the answer.

Meditate, don't medicate.

Ditto for muscle relaxants—they don't really relax muscles that are in spasm. They work more on the central nervous system, or brain. Again, the effect is temporary, and they can have some depressive side effects that are an enemy of recovery from back ailments.

We're now being told that, in general, physi-

cians in the medical community undertreat pain, and therefore it has been established as a fifth vital sign, after blood pressure, breathing, pulse, and body temperature. Patients with excruciating back pain are a thorny problem for doctors. On the one hand, doctors are committed to providing relief; on the other, they're wary about causing a serious addiction. The issue is further complicated by the fact that we all respond differently to pain and have varying tolerances for it, and there's a very deep emotional component involved. One of my colleagues, a British chap, is fond of saying, "The pine in the spine is minely in the brine." He's quite right about the role of the brain in health, as we've covered at some length herein.

"The pine in the spine is minely in the brine."

I always draw that fine line between being compassionate and sentencing someone to a lifetime of narcotic use. Some very smart people believe you can easily get caught up in that kind of situation, and they're right. My friend and colleague Nick Shamie, MD, is a prominent spine surgeon and UCLA School of Medicine professor, and he has some pointed thoughts about prescription drug abuse:

Pain is the body's signal that alerts the patient that something is wrong. This is helpful because the patient will seek care before the condition becomes more serious, and it helps the physician to locate the problem.

But if the source of the pain is not treated and only masked with pain medications, the condition can progress and cause more serious irreversible damage to tissues that will be hard to treat. Pain med-seeking behavior can also arise by improper/excessive or prolonged prescription of pain medications and modalities, redirecting the patient's focus from "trying to get better" to "trying to get more pain meds"—one definition of drug addiction.

Pain medications are good for short-term care until the source of the problem is discovered and properly treated. A problem arises when patients with acute pain seek help from "pain specialists" who at times have very little training in discovering and treating the source of pain. This problem is especially noted in spine patients because most spine surgeons refer patients to pain management colleagues until surgery is necessary. The pain medication administration is prolonged in this scenario and can be detrimental to proper diagnosis and treatment.

You simply must be on guard against over-medicating. Take a pill at the onset of a back problem if you absolutely must, but your priority should be finding a reputable medical practice that is interested in making you better rather than having you come back. If all they're doing is numbing you without addressing the stress and emotional issues and the root cause of your problem, if they're just treating the pain without looking at the whole picture, you're in the wrong place.

THE RIGHT PLACES TO BE

After decades spent as an orthopaedic specialist, supplemented liberally with continu-

BACK STORY

Even the Laser Spine Institute (LSI), a national group of high-tech surgeons specializing in minimally invasive endoscopic spinal surgery, has come to realize the importance of the non-surgical approaches to back pain. LSI recently acquired Aspen Back & Body (founded by Clint Phillips and located in Aspen, Colorado), a high-end destination spa specializing exclusively in spinal health, wellness, and recovery. They offer innovative multi-disciplinary, individualized programs. Clearly a one- to three-week stay in Aspen is not for everyone, but they do have educational videos, and their philosophy is right—you need a comprehensive mind-body approach, and a qualified support team around you, to create a personalized program including lifestyle modification that will become an integral part of your life going forward. Take the time and effort to assemble your own local team of caring professionals.

ing education, I have no doubt in my mind about how to maintain a healthy frame. And even though, as I said earlier, I don't have all the answers when it comes to out-of-whack backs, I do know that you can find what you need for your chronic back ailment among the numerous and diverse approaches that are readily available to you. Because everyone is unique, a certain amount of the trial and error that we discussed in Step 2 is to be expected here. Certain approaches, and certain options within an approach, will prove to be better suited to your case. You'll find them as long as you keep searching.

You should know, too, that most problem-atic cases are going to require more than one option to secure relief. Resist the hope that you'll find the Holy Grail in one office, because the reality is that multiple, coordinated treatments are the rule rather than the exception, especially in the more chronic situations. Be wary of anyone who claims to have *the* solution, and of anyone who is reluctant to work in conjunction with other professionals. Investigate the modalities below and don't give up on one until you're sure it doesn't have any promise for you. (This might require visiting more than one specialist in a given area, because styles, personalities, skill, and experience vary. What one person couldn't do for you, another just might be able to.) Along the way, stick with those whose sole focus is on helping you get well as soon as possible—whatever it takes.

PAIN SPECIALISTS

When pain is acute and it won't let up, you won't be able to think about anything else or do anything else to get on the path that will solve the problem long term. Pain must therefore be addressed, but its treatment must include pain management along with pain elimination.

There is so much in the media telling us not to suffer any pain at all that we have become obsessed with the removal of every discomfort from our lives. Honesty demands that doctors inform their patients that drugs alone aren't the answer, that a certain amount of ache is to be expected on the road to recovery, and that there are sequential options in the armamentarium for dealing with pain.

MEDICATION

If you showed up in my office in extreme pain, I would never deny you the drugs you need—temporarily.

Let me say that again: temporarily. If the first line of defense—OTC (over-the-counter) acetaminophen (such as Tylenol) and ibuprofen (such as Advil)—doesn't provide enough relief after the specific time period noted on their bottles, your doctor has many options, some of which can be administered via the new patches that release measured doses over time to improve effectiveness.

- **Muscle relaxers** such as diazepam (Valium). I'm not a big fan for reasons already noted.

- **Antidepressants:** These drugs block pain messages on their way to the brain and can help increase production of endorphins, your body's natural painkillers.

- **Anticonvulsants:** Prescription medication like Neurontin and Lyrica (both anti-seizure medicines) can positively affect nerve function in ways that dampen and relieve nerve-related pain.

- **Opioids:** In the most extreme cases, your doctor will prescribe and carefully monitor the use of narcotics such as hydrocodone (Vicodin), oxycodone (Percocet), codeine, meperidine (Demerol), or morphine.

Every option has serious side effects, so do your due diligence by discussing it in depth before you put anything into your body. And think "short term" rather than longer use or final answer.

■ TRACTION

This modality applies gentle force to stretch and mobilize the spine to alleviate back pain and spasm. Despite recent advances such as computer-controlled machines, the jury is still out about the merits of this treatment. Regardless, the truth is some patients have found relief this way, so it should be part of the discussion. (Being hospitalized for traction, something that *was* very common a few years back during my orthopaedic training, is absolutely not warranted, because traction can be tried in most physical therapy outpatient settings.)

■ SPINAL INJECTIONS

As a last resort, your pain specialist can recommend:

■ An epidural steroid to relieve pinched nerve roots in the lower back. These injections can now be targeted to very specific inflamed or pinched nerve roots.

■ A sympathetic nerve block, targeting the nerves that control some of your body's involuntary functions, such as the opening and closing of blood vessels.

■ Facet joint numbing and inflammation reduction with a combination of an anesthetic and cortisone.

■ A spinal cord stimulator to block pain signals.

The above are last resorts for good reason. They're tricky, they can't be used over the long term, and they relieve pain only in a relatively small percentage of people with back pain. Find a specialist—often an anesthesiologist or physiatrist—with a great reputation, good judgment, and a gentle hand.

For advice regarding the need for spinal injections, I usually turn to Larry Chou, MD, of Premier Orthopaedics. He is a wonderful, caring physician who knows the spine inside and out. Here are his thoughts:

"Low back pain is virtually ubiquitous, yet only a limited number of people

BACK STORY

MedX lumbar rehabilitation has helped many of my patients with lower back pain for when virtually every other treatment option has failed. In my area, I am fortunate to have Main Line Medical Exercise, pioneered by Roger Schwab and one of the most experienced MedX centers in the world. Unlike other muscles in the body, the important lumbar extension muscles (the key to a healthy, durable spine) can be very difficult to isolate. MedX does just that in a unique way and also can be used to strengthen spinal rotation.

undergo a spinal injection for pain relief and even fewer consider surgical options. A spinal injection can be very useful for both diagnostic purposes (localizing the source of pain or "pain generator") and therapeutic purposes (for pain relief). Potential sources of pain include the disks, spinal joints, and spinal nerves, among others. A spinal injection is never required, but rather, it should be considered when one's pain sufficiently interferes with function, e.g., work, play, sleep, exercise, or psychological well-being. As long as the pain can be considered 'tolerable,' then spinal injections can be deferred."

■ PHYSICAL THERAPISTS

After you and your doctor have stanched your acute pain, it's time to move on. Your next stop, with or without some pain that remains, is a visit with a reputable biomechanical specialist who works closely with your orthopaedic doctor or spine specialist.

The evidence is overwhelming that physical therapy (PT) as it is practiced best today helps you not only get past a crisis but also avoid a recurrence. The latest reports are that it is better than medical care alone—and better than chiropractic. A literature study published in the February 2009 issue of the *Journal of the American Academy of Orthopaedic Surgeons* revealed that the most effective treatment for lower back pain is a combination of PT and anti-inflammatory medication (hence the need to work closely with a medical doctor). Specifics of that study include the following that are of great import:

■ Ninety percent of patients will see their lower back symptoms fade within 3 months.

■ Most patients will recover within 6 weeks.

- PT that focuses on strengthening core muscle groups has demonstrated positive effects in patients with disk-related pain.

- Educating patients on better body mechanics lessens the strain placed on the lumbar region.

The best physical therapists use the McKenzie Method, which we talked about in Step 2 and which also categorizes patients by their mechanical response to pain. The most common group is those who feel pain in a concentrated area when bending in a particular direction, known as derangement. A second category, dysfunction, is composed of those who feel pain in conjunction with a limited range of motion. Those who feel pain at the end of a range of motion make up the postural category. (Some patients have a combination of the above.) When your therapist knows what's going on, he or she can administer the right treatments.

HEAT OR ICE

You'll be amazed at the difference professional-grade pads and packs make. Relief can be immediate, and you'll be able to be more active sooner than you think.

ULTRASOUND

This approach delivers energy deeper into the body than heating pads are able to do. Any pain relief it provides results from increased bloodflow to the injured area.

"STIM" UNITS

I have found two modalities for muscle and/or nerve stimulation particularly helpful and effective. H-Wave is a unique neuromuscular stimulator that can reduce pain and spasm, and through a variety of biochemical and cellular processes it can promote healing. InterX is an interactive handheld neuro-stim device that acts like acupuncture without needles. (These particular units are used widely by athletic trainers and physical therapists working with professional and higher-level athletes to keep them going.)

TENS is a different type of stim unit that can help with pain relief in some cases, but is more time-intensive. I prefer the use of H-Wave and/or InterX to quiet the pain so that you can get mobile and get moving with your exercise program.

BACK STORY

Champ L. Baker Jr., MD, during his term as president of the American Orthopaedic Society for Sports Medicine (AOSSM), used the following short history of medicine to put health care in perspective.

2000 BC: Here, eat this root.

AD 1600: That root is heathen. Here, say this prayer.

AD 1850: That prayer is superstition. Here, drink this potion.

AD 1940: That potion is snake oil. Here, swallow this pill.

AD 1985: That pill is ineffective. Here, take this antibiotic.

AD 2000: That antibiotic doesn't work anymore. Here, eat this root.

Dr. Champ wasn't eschewing high-tech advances in medicine. He was just making the point that sometimes going back to our "roots," as represented by alternative healers, can, indeed, result in a partial, if not complete, cure.

■ CONTROLLED EXERCISE

Your therapist has a host of options to get your lower back frame oiled up. If your case is severe, he or she might start with just some pain-relieving modalities and simple stretches in your first few sessions. Then you'll move on to other exercises that will include some of those in this book. Each one will be explained in detail, how it works your affected area and how it should be carefully performed. To get the desired improvement, it's imperative that each exercise is performed precisely. There will be some trial and error as to which movements might be best for you at your particular stage of recovery. After a little guidance from your therapist, you'll be able to do them on your own, and your technique and progress will be checked in subsequent sessions.

Isolating the lumbar muscles for evaluation and treatment was a huge problem until Arthur Jones, the inventor of Nautilus machines, developed the MedX line of equipment. Your "cheatin' bod" finds ways to accommodate physical restrictions that result from injury, and may lean unnaturally using the buttocks or hamstrings, instead of isolating your lower back muscles, which are designed to do the work the right way. A MedX evaluation will show that most people with chronic back pain have problems with strength and endurance in their lower back extensor muscles. Work on those properly, and the odds are you'll resolve your backache.

The PT options will ease your pain and then teach you how to avoid certain movements that aggravate your condition. (A common one is rotating hips while seated instead of turning the chair.) Many even offer a "back school" program (see page 154) geared to teach you everything about maintaining a healthy lower back as well as navigating the world when your back is not being very cooperative.

Once you've learned to control things, you'll be gradually introduced to more extensive routines while nurturing your lower back muscles, your abs, your intra-pelvic musculature, or your hamstrings. If you're the average patient with a lower

BACK STORY

Recent scientific studies have shown reproducible brain localized response to acupuncture when using advanced functional magnetic resonance imaging (MRI). I personally witnessed some amazing work with acupuncture and other Eastern modalities when I was part of a month-long sports medicine exchange to China in the 1980s, before the term *alternative medicine* was coined. So if you're frustrated, acupuncture might be worth a try.

back ailment, you will only need a few weeks of assisted therapy before you'll be able to use a home exercise program on your own. You may need to check in with your therapist now and then, however, to stay on track.

And you should know that many certified athletic trainers (ATCs) offer similar exercise and preventive routines, especially to sports teams on high school, college, and professional levels.

■ PSYCHIATRISTS AND PSYCHOLOGISTS

If you've been paying attention, you know that the mind is as important in frame health as it is in general health. Having input from highly recommended professional counselors is valuable from the start of recovery or at any time during it, and it is a must if every other option has been exhausted—it just might be that your head is getting in the way of your back somehow.

ALTERNATIVE HEALERS

According to the US Department of Health and Human Services, 38 percent of adults (about *90 million* of us) used some form of complementary or alternative medicine (CAM) in 2005. If medical doctors and almighty surgeons are honest, they acknowledge the fact that nontraditional health-care disciplines have had proven merit for pain management in many cases and are no doubt worth a try for those who have been dealing with pain for an extended period.

I believe that no one has all of the answers and sometimes you have to reach out to other people—whether it's an acupuncturist or deep-tissue therapist or massage therapist or chiropractor—and let them do what they can do for you. My mind opened to this in the early 1980s, before the word *alternative* was attached to *medicine.* The majority of people back then held a dim view of nontraditional health-care practitioners and saw the whole group as quacks prac-

ticing chicanery. When I started working with professional and Olympic athletes who almost always used massage therapists and chiropractors, my eyes opened wide. I saw the frame healing they delivered that enabled their patients to maintain extreme levels of activity. I spent 25-plus years working with professional dancers at the Pennsylvania Ballet, who were some of the first to open my eyes to things like the Alexander Technique and Pilates. Eventually, as you know, I got to experience some alternative healing myself when my good friend Neil Liebman laid some chiropractic on me.

So we'll start the discussion of "alternative" alternatives with a little bit more about that specialty, and then move on to other modalities that don't have a lot of research backing them up. But even if reports of success are only anecdotal, I've seen with my own eyes how just about all of them helped some people. Bottom line? Relief is all that matters, and you could finally find yours among the possibilities that follow.

▪ CHIROPRACTIC

We talked about it in Step 2, so if you haven't tried that yet, by all means give it a whirl. It's well accepted for occasional, short-term relief, and it is the most common alternative therapy, chosen by about 15 percent of the population every year. In addition to spinal manipulation, your therapist might also use ultrasound or electrical stimulation as well as these techniques.

- **Trigger point therapy:** Hypertonic (tight) painful points are identified and released via direct finger pressure.

- **Graston technique:** This soft-tissue mobilization therapy uses repeated strokes of instruments developed in 1987 by David Graston, a machinist by trade, that research has shown increase the number of fibroblasts (special cells that help heal injury).

- **Active release techniques** (**ART**): This therapy is geared to improve muscle and tendon function and healing.

- **Machine-assisted massage:** Devices like the ArthoStim and a variety of percussors provide deep stimulation to free up moving parts.

If chiropractic wasn't of much help to you, it might be worth trying it with another practitioner. The connection may prove much better with different hands on your frame. If you go this

route, make sure you work with a chiropractor who coordinates treatment with your regular physician.

- **MASSAGE THERAPY**

A recent study of medical literature showed that this approach decreases symptoms and improves function in patients with nonspecific lower back pain, especially when it is used in conjunction with exercise and education.

- **ACUPUNCTURE**

Some experts suggest that the fine needles used for this treatment overload certain nerve centers, or "Chi points," to block transmission of nerve impulses. Researchers aren't sure how much physical versus psychological benefit it delivers, but acupuncture has worked in many cases, and it's relatively safe. I am a believer.

ACUPRESSURE

This modality works along the same lines as acupuncture, except practitioners use their thumbs, fingers, and elbows to target specific Chi points. Reflexology, which concentrates pressure on the hands and feet, is a subcategory here.

BACK SCHOOLS

These are not buildings—they're programs that promote understanding of how the spine functions, how to protect it in daily life, and how you can live with compromises. Do you have an ergonomic chair, and is it the right height? Do you need a footrest? Are you flexible enough? When you "graduate," you'll know a lot about ergonomics— how your body interacts with the environment. You'll know how to maintain good posture and how to sit, walk, drive, and travel on public transportation to navigate daily life and stay out of back trouble.

YOGA

Our stress-filled lives exacerbate injuries and prolong recovery. To get off the "treadmill," you might try these mind-body exercises to slow down your thought processes and body reactions. They emphasize muscle balance, providing restorative benefit in some cases.

BIOFEEDBACK

This is a process that enables you to learn how to change physiological activity to improve health and performance. It has been used with some success for ADD/ADHD, headaches, and chronic pain. For back ailments, the practitioner teaches you mental and physical exercises that are monitored by sensors applied to specific points on your body to gauge physiological response. The theory is that, over time, muscle memory will take over and ensure proper movement of body parts. You can learn to not only relax your mind and lower your blood pressure but also relax and "short-circuit" muscles that are chronically misbehaving, locked in spasm.

HANDS-ON

The healing effect of the "laying on of hands" can't be proven, but it usually provides some psychological impact, giving you the confidence to move on to other therapies. If you're in Step 6, you have to try *anything* that might help.

You've probably noted that education

BACK STORY

has been mentioned a couple of times. It's a huge part of recovery, so never stop trying to learn what will work for you.

MORE HELPFUL HINTS

There are some relatively minor things you should explore because they could have a major impact on the speed or ease of recovery. The following could be part of your overall plan for lower back recovery:

▪ SPINAL SUPPORTS

While there is no evidence in the medical literature to support long-term use of a flexible, rigid, or semi-rigid back brace or corset, it might provide temporary relief by limiting motion and/or stabilizing weak or injured frame members. I believe that supports provide a reminder to use your back more correctly. The neoprene ones also make you sweat underneath, keeping the lower back muscles "warmed up" and thus less vulnerable to strain. The trick here is to use it correctly, and only for a short while so you don't develop a psychological dependency on it that prevents you from doing other exercises that lead to more lasting relief. A support can also be helpful for individuals transitioning back to sports or labor-intensive jobs.

▪ BEDTIME

You spend up to a third of your life asleep, so it's always important to support your frame properly in bed, and it's critical when you have a back injury. As I mentioned earlier, I prefer a semi-firm but accommodating pillow-topped mattress, and you should ask

BACK STORY

The lower back program that I designed for myself first was life altering for me. I had been worried about being able to raise my kids and play with them and someday walk them down the aisle. I'd had weeks where I just couldn't walk right and some nights when I would just toss and turn until the sun came up. And there were times when my back was so out of whack that I'd have to lean on something whenever I stood up.

I can go out and play a pretty high level of tennis now without getting into too much trouble, but I still endure some back episodes when I pick up something in the closet or reach for my son when he darts or jumps suddenly. But whenever I have pain, I know I can work through it. If it's really uncomfortable, I'll take some Tylenol or Aleve to just lower the pain level to the point where I might be able to do some stretching, walking, or bike riding. I won't do provocative exercises, but I will do those movement patterns that I think will help me. If I'm really bad off, I'll call my trusty chiropractor pal Neil Liebman and have him work his magic. Then I get right back to the routines in Step 5 to recover my frame and make it stronger so my lower back episodes will be further apart, less severe, and easier to recover from.

your doctor or therapist for directions on sleep positions (on the stomach is usually inadvisable for lower back pain) and about investing in an adjustable bed that might ease the load on your troubled area.

■ SUPPLEMENTS

As I mentioned previously, I am a big believer that what you put in your mouth affects your frame, for better or worse.

This is true of nutritional choices as well as certain vitamins and supplements. The joint supplements glucosamine and chondroitin sulfate are helpful for individuals with osteoarthritis, especially in the knee and hip. It is not unusual for certain spine problems (both lower back and neck) to have an element of wear-and-tear arthritis. And for those patients I strongly recommend a 2-month trial of a high-quality joint supplement. The brand that I have the most faith in, and use personally, is Cosamin by Nutramax Labs. For years I have used Cosamin DS, but I've recently switched to the newer Cosamin ASU, which has the same glucosamine/chondroitin blend but also includes soy, avocado, and green tea extract, all very useful in fighting inflammation and protecting your joints, even the little ones deep in your spine.

■ LIFESTYLE MODIFICATIONS

Most of us take the way we live for granted as we go about the day's activities. Revisit the BLT and posture recommendations in Step 1 and check with your chiropractor or physical therapist to be absolutely certain you aren't doing something unconsciously that isn't helping you.

And then there may be an issue about what you do for a living. Cumulative trauma disorder (CTD) results from:

- ■ Repetitive movements with little force (such as carpal tunnel syndrome)

- ■ Less repetitive but more forceful movements (such as tennis elbow)

- ■ Large loads without movement

It just might be that your work is contributing to your backache or hampering progress toward recovery, so discuss it in detail with the professionals on your team. If necessary, pull out all the stops to modify your job or environment. Maybe you could switch from physical labor to a desk job (maybe just temporarily), or vice versa, or reduce the physical stresses that cause or add to problems. You won't know until you have an honest discussion with your bosses and coworkers.

Take a hard look at all of your daily activities and routines to find any area that could ease your trauma and open up a path to recovery. And don't overlook your sex life when you do. (If your pain is severe, it would probably be a good idea to avoid sex for a short time, but sexual activity has systemwide benefits for both the mind and the body, and it keeps relationships healthy as well. As soon as your pain subsides, you should communicate any limitations you have to your partner and work with him or her to find the positions and options that work best for you. Incorporate warm showers and massage as part of the fun in making new discoveries together.)

PRAYER

The "anything" above includes this option. I'm fond of saying, "Meditate, don't medicate," and it doesn't matter whether you use yoga, communing with nature, or spirituality of one type or denomination or another. I'm not here to convert anyone, and I'll admit that prayer is not usually first on the doctor's prescription pad. But I will say that by whatever name it's called, prayer has been shown on many occasions to have a significant salutary effect.

PAIN VERSUS A PRODUCTIVE LIFE

There are so many people who have chronic back pain, and some are a complete wreck. They just have it, they've tried and tried to find relief—maybe have even had one or more surgeries—and they feel there's nothing anybody can do. Physical problems often lead to psychological decline, and that's a dangerous combination.

I'm here to tell you that no matter what state your back is in, there are still some ways to improve your condition. Even if you've tried

everything in these pages, there's more you can do—salvage some hope and try some approaches again, or find another doctor who has a different perspective on your case or has different colleagues to recommend, or combines therapies in a different way. The Resources section at the end of this book is a good place to start if you are stymied.

If it's there, it's there—but that doesn't mean you can't focus on something other than your pain and reap the benefit of getting something worthwhile accomplished. At the very least, it'll distract you from the ache that nags at you, and your mind will be refreshed. I know if you're out there doing something, being productive, managing your stress, having a better outlook on life, not feeling like a victim, always looking at what you can do, not at what you can't do, you'll make progress. It might be humbling at first, but you've got to start somewhere.

You simply must "reframe" your problem. Unless you are slated for back surgery, whatever pain you have can be managed. See it in a new light, as professional athletes do all the time, and understand the difference between pain and injury, between hurt and harm. If you're not going to cause additional harm (that's the difference between just having discomfort or pain and making an injury worse),

BACK STORY

My friend and colleague Todd Albert is a very talented and renowned spine surgeon who had patients stacked up at the Philadelphia hospital where he operates, but he'd gotten to the point where he wasn't sure how many people he was helping with surgery. He feels more and more that doing all of the less drastic things to strengthen the back before resorting to the knife is more often the way to go, and his practice has evolved toward biomechanical treatment and prevention. He figures (and I concur) that, at the very least, framework will improve the speed and quality of recovery.

you've got to steel yourself and work through it. A lot of times you have pain and you think because it hurts, you're going to harm yourself if you do anything. In the overriding majority of cases, that just isn't so.

With my back problem, I resist the urge to feel sorry for myself, and I find that diving into surgery or clinical procedures when I am in the midst of an episode helps not only my patients who need me but also my condition. When I take the focus off my back, I give my body a chance to recover on its own. It's not a fluke—it happens to me just about every time, and I've seen it time and time again with many patients. "Leave your body" for a time, and you might be another one who asks, "Where did that kink go?"

Remember always that you are far from alone in your quest. Those near and dear to you will do anything they can for you. And, if you never give up, you'll assemble a few talented health-care professionals who will help you.

ALL FOR ONE AND . . . ALL FOR ONE

You're the first member of the team whose combined efforts are required to restore your frame health. Once you've made the (renewed?) commitment to yourself to get better, recruit anyone else who can make a difference. It takes more than an orthopaedic surgeon or a neurologist in almost every tough case, and many conventional doctors aren't open to alternative care. If it takes breaking some ties, so be it. The end result of having a couple of committed individuals on your side is all that matters. You want a team that's "got your back."

If you're saddled with a long-term back ailment, the collaborative approach is the way to go. An enlightened practitioner would welcome a discussion about any information in these pages that you think could be a factor in your case. If you're not satisfied with answers to your questions, move on to someone else. I've had the honor and privilege of knowing and working with countless gifted and capable professionals all over the world; there are plenty to choose from everywhere. Find yours, and do the work that needs to be done together.

ACTIVE FOR LIFE

If you fail to manage your pain, you will have severe physical restrictions, and there is also evidence that suggests long-term pain may age your brain prematurely. In a Northwestern University study involving 52 people, the average size of the thalamus (the region associated with decision making and social behavior) was up to 11 percent smaller in the 26 people with chronic back pain.

Such a reduction is equivalent to that which occurs after 10 or 20 years of normal aging. Any way you look at it, you have to change course and head back to a healthy frame.

For the last time (at least in this book)—being sedentary is not an option. There is much to investigate, not the least of which are some directed exercises for your out-of-whack back. Do your due diligence and "draft" your team of professionals who have the requisite skills to help you conquer your back pain. Get the recommendations you need from doctors and other people you trust, especially if they are or have been personally acquainted with back trouble. Interview any practitioner you are considering as you would a new babysitter; check credentials and references, and make sure only the latest equipment and techniques will be used on you. Explore your options methodically, use trial and error to discover the Rosetta stone that works for you, and stick to it for as long as it takes.

You've spent a lot of time with your aches, and it might take some time before you make significant progress. But if you think out of the box, you *will* get out of that box you're in.

You can, indeed, end back pain *now*.

AFTERWORD

When I wrote *FrameWork* a few years ago, artificial disks were only being considered—now they're being put in necks and backs on a regular basis. That doesn't mean you're a candidate for one and should run to the nearest OR, but it is reassuring to know that medicine advances as time does. In the blink of an eye, technology is advancing at warp speed; treatments and interventions I never thought possible during my surgical training years ago are now either here or just on the horizon.

The years between 2000 and 2010 have been designated as the Bone and Joint Decade, and the world of orthopaedics is booming right now. The most exciting development is that we're getting past the concept of repair and moving into regeneration. It's not just about patching things up; it's about rebuilding, getting a new start with new body parts that, more and more, come from your own cells instead of a factory. This was once the stuff of science fiction, and the fact that it is only one part of the new armamentarium for treating back pain makes the future bright, indeed.

Surgical Advances

"Watch one, do one, teach one" is the cornerstone of surgical education. Doctors worth their salt never stop learning and never stop discovering, so major progress in procedures and equipment seems to occur almost daily in one place or another. Coming soon to a "theater" near you:

■ **REVOLUTIONARY TECHNIQUES**
Surgeries are being performed via smaller and smaller incisions. Minimally invasive surgery (MIS), which has become popular in hip and knee replacement or reconstruction surgeries, is now also being used in spinal surgery. MIS results in less pain, shorter hospitalizations, and overall quicker recovery.

■ **COMPUTERS IN THE OR**
Digital technology has found a rightful place in the surgical suite. Computer-

BACK STORY

"If I hold off a few years, are there better treatments coming?" This is a question I hear from my patients all the time. They're savvy and want to know what doctors, technicians, and researchers are going to come up with next, what's going to be different down the road, because there's always something new over the next hill or around the next bend. I can assure you that whether it's for knees or hips or backs, medical laboratories, offices, hospitals—and classrooms—are abuzz with activity and hope for the next breakthrough. The future is indeed bright.

assisted spinal navigation and image guidance allows for better visualization of surgical anatomy and more accurate placement of instruments and fixation devices such as screws. Also, don't be surprised if a robot similar to one commonly used for prostate surgery assists in your surgery—that modality is being used more and more in orthopaedics and neurosurgery. The use of robots has also opened the doors for remote surgery, where an expert from another city or state, or even somewhere else in the world, can assist with or perform your surgery!

■ **HIGH-TECH ALPHABET SOUP**

MIS, TLIF, PLIF, ALIF, XLIF, TDR— what looks like a word jumble or cryptogram is actually a group of acronyms commonly seen in the schedule in most spine surgery conferences. They refer to new technologies and new instrumentation to repair and stabilize problem spines. You may hear about dynamic stabilizing devices or motion preservation technologies, both of which try to maintain a more normal functioning mobile spine. Surgeons are now able to preserve mobility in some cases with a TDR (total disk replacement) rather than fuse the segment via ALIF (anterior lumbar interbody fusion) or PLIF (posterior lumbar interbody fusion).

Regenerated Disks and Bones

There is a tremendous amount of research in the use of biologics (blood, blood components, vaccines, allergenics, somatic cells, gene therapy, and recombinant therapeutic proteins) as it relates to the spine. Substances that enhance bone formation can help patients who need to undergo spinal fusion. Instead of having to utilize bone graft taken from the patient's own body, with larger or extra incisions and increased risk of pain and/or bleeding, bone graft substitutes are being utilized to create new bone and aid with the fusion process. Bone morphogenic proteins (BMP) and growth factors like rhGDF-5 (recombinant human growth and differentiation factor-5) are being used experimentally to enhance fusion rates, but there have been some reports of higher complication rates with BMPs when used in spinal fusion, so clinical use is not widespread yet.

Research is also being done on biologic agents to repair, or even regenerate, injured or degenerated intervertebral disks. Mesenchymal stem cells also have the potential to regenerate disks, and they can do likewise for bone and cartilage. They show real promise for giving damaged knees, hips, and spines a new start.

Also, human embryonic stem cells are now being studied as a means to improve nerve function and recovery after serious spinal cord injury with paralysis. Regenerating damaged nerves may be just around the corner, and when it is available, it will clearly have a place in the world of spine care.

BACK STORY

Getting Back on Their Feet, a DVD by Richard Longland (www.arthropatient.org), is a wonderful documentary that follows seven patients through their struggles and successes with back surgery, with an emphasis on disk replacement. Longland, a disk replacement recipient himself, portrays the complexities of lower back care, nonoperative and operative alike, including the toll it takes on individuals' lives. I recommend this DVD to anyone suffering with chronic lower back pain, especially those contemplating any type of lower back surgery.

Disk Replacement

An artificial disk (prosthesis) can be implanted into the spine in an attempt to simulate the function of a normal disk. It is made from metal or plasticlike polymer materials, or a combination of the two. Results have been very promising, allowing for more normal spine function. Disk replacement is not suitable for all patients with back pain, as select criteria must be met.

BACK STORY

I recently had the opportunity to ask Todd Albert, MD, about his thoughts on the most exciting emergent technologies for lower back surgical care. Dr. Albert, a renowned spine surgeon, is chairman of orthopaedic surgery at the Rothman Institute in Philadelphia. Here are his very positive thoughts about the future of spine surgery and spinal care: "The most exciting developments are the new motion-sparing technologies, the bone growth factors and molecules that help us with fusion so that we don't have to take bone graft from patients, and regenerative technologies for the disk using stem cells and other methodologies which are on the horizon. In terms of minimally invasive care, the stem cell technologies noted above are likely to be able to be used with injection techniques and minimally invasive techniques so a patient barely has to go into the hospital to obtain these treatments to regenerate the disk. Also exciting are the diagnostic modalities and the tests for diagnosing genetic predisposition to lower back pain complaints."

Gene Therapy

This cutting-edge process involves the transfer of an appropriate gene into a cell, via a viral or nonviral "vector," to prevent degenerative disk disease, regenerate degenerated disks, and promote spinal fusion, allowing the body to heal itself.

PATIENT-CENTERED CARE AND THE PAIN GAME

All too often a surgeon is happy, but the patient is not. The wound has healed beautifully, the x-rays look terrific, the fusion is solid—but the patient is still not functioning as well as he or she expected. A mismatch in expectations between the doctor and the patient occurs.

The news that adds to future promise is that medical professionals have become much more in tune with seeing things from the patient's viewpoint and strive for both happy x-rays and happy, satisfied patients. Surgeons are trying harder to be not only "high tech" but also "high touch." More and more research is considering the patient's viewpoint, function, and satisfaction. Armed with that knowledge, physicians are getting better at seeing things through the patient's eyes.

The program in this book is patient-centered and is suitable for those who have either avoided or needed surgery. As always, however, check with your doctor to assure that anything herein you want to incorporate is right for you.

I've acknowledged a couple of times in these pages that pain is a challenging, often misleading friend and foe for those who have back problems. Physicians want to soothe pain but don't want to create additional problems for their patients. They're constantly pulled in opposite directions: Medicate or not? And for how long? Not easy questions when dealing with a condition that can be chronic and/or recurrent, the hallmarks of back pain.

Science is just beginning to understand the individual variation in pain susceptibility and intensity. Although areas like patient outcomes and pain management are not as sexy as artificial disks and regenerated nerves, research in these areas is extremely important and will help many patients in the years to come. Doctors of every stripe are constantly looking for better pain medications that do not have dependence and addiction potential, and for better modalities for delivery such as patches or specialized injec-

tions directly into the damaged areas. Our search for knowledge includes the painstaking work of researchers like Kenneth Blum, PhD, at the University of Florida, who is shedding light on the genetic factors that may predispose some to addictive behaviors. That could lead to new options for compassionate management of pain for those more susceptible to addiction.

LOOKING AHEAD

Even if nothing in the six steps here works quite right for you, there's plenty on the horizon. Don't panic, don't give up hope, because there's a lot going on and the next discovery or innovation that passes scrutiny might just be the one that solves your back problem once and for all.

The message here is you've got to hold on. If you keep searching, you will find something that helps you. Do the best you can to manage your back condition, keep researching, always learn as doctors do, and never stop trying new things. The future may not be now for you, but it's not that far away. And it wouldn't surprise me at all if some "futuristic" back treatments are a reality by the time the next entry in the *FrameWork* "Active for Life" Series hits the shelves.

ADDITIONAL RESOURCES

WEB SITES

www.aaos.org (American Academy of Orthopaedic Surgeons)

www.acatoday.org (American Chiropractic Association)

www.apta.org (American Physical Therapy Association)

www.arthropatient.org (Arthroplasty Patient Foundation)

www.DrNick.com (Nicholas A. DiNubile, MD)

www.DrWeil.com (Andrew Weil, MD, alternative medicine)

www.nih.gov (National Institutes of Health)

www.orthoinfo.org (AAOS—Your Orthopaedic Connection)

www.spine.org (North American Spine Society)

www.spine-health.com (Spine-Health)

www.spineuniverse.com (SpineUniverse)

www.spri.com

BOOKS

FrameWork by Nicholas A. DiNubile, MD, with William Patrick (Rodale Inc., 2005)

Healing Back Pain: The Mind-Body Connection by John E. Sarno, MD (Warner Books, 1991)

Healing Moves by Carol Krucoff and Mitchell Krucoff (Healthy Learning, 2009)

Low Back Disorders by Stuart McGill (Human Kinetics, 2007)

Rothman-Simeone The Spine, edited by Harry Herkowitz, MD (Saunders, 2006)

Treat Your Own Back by Robin A. McKenzie (Orthopaedic Physical Therapy Product, 1997)

Ultimate Back Fitness and Performance by Stuart McGill (Stuart McGill, 2004)

DVDS

Getting Back on Their Feet by Richard Longland (Arthroplasty Patient Foundation—www.arthropatient.org)

Heal the Back with Dr. Clinton G. Phillips (Aspen Back and Body—www.aspenback.com)

Mayo Clinic Wellness Solutions for Back Pain with Dr. Brent A. Bauer, Dr. Randy A. Shelerud, and yoga master Rodney Yee (Mayo Clinic/Gaiam)

Your Body's FrameWork, with Dr. Nick DiNubile, as seen originally on PBS (Santa Fe Productions, Inc.)

Your Body's FrameWork Home WorkOut by Nicholas A. DiNubile, MD (Santa Fe Productions, Inc.)

Your Client: FrameWork (for fitness professionals and personal trainers) by Nicolas A. DiNubile, MD (American Council on Exercise—www.acefitness.org)

PRODUCTS

H-Wave.com (neuromuscular stimulation)

NRG-unlimited.com (InterX nerve stimulator)

NutramaxLabs.com (joint supplements)

SPRI Home *FrameWork* Low Back Fitness Products (www.spri.com)

Interchangeable tubing system

Interchangeable tubing system attachments

(interchangeable handle and/or dual hand strap)

Stability Ball (Xercise Balls)

Xergym door attachment

Xertube

ABOUT THE AUTHORS

NICHOLAS A. DiNUBILE, MD, an orthopaedic surgeon specializing in sports medicine and a best-selling author, has served as orthopaedic consultant to the Philadelphia 76ers and the Pennsylvania Ballet. His advice has been featured on prime-time television and in the *New York Times*, the *Wall Street Journal*, the *Washington Post*, and *Newsweek*. His award-winning television special, *Your Body's FrameWork*, has been aired on PBS nationwide. Learn more about Dr. DiNubile at DrNick.com.

BRUCE SCALI writes across multiple genres and transforms complex subject matter to make it accessible to every reader.

INDEX

Boldface page references indicate photographs. <u>Underscored</u> references indicate boxed text.